Selling

Selling Yoga

*From Counterculture
to Pop Culture*

ANDREA R. JAIN

OXFORD
UNIVERSITY PRESS

OXFORD
UNIVERSITY PRESS

Oxford University Press is a department of the University of Oxford.
It furthers the University's objective of excellence in research, scholarship,
and education by publishing worldwide.

Oxford   New York
Auckland   Cape Town   Dar es Salaam   Hong Kong   Karachi
Kuala Lumpur   Madrid   Melbourne   Mexico City   Nairobi
New Delhi   Shanghai   Taipei   Toronto

With offices in
Argentina   Austria   Brazil   Chile   Czech Republic   France   Greece
Guatemala   Hungary   Italy   Japan   Poland   Portugal   Singapore
South Korea   Switzerland   Thailand   Turkey   Ukraine   Vietnam

Oxford is a registered trademark of Oxford University Press
in the UK and certain other countries.

Published in the United States of America by
Oxford University Press
198 Madison Avenue, New York, NY 10016

© Oxford University Press 2015

Library of Congress Cataloging-in-Publication Data
Jain, Andrea R., author.
Selling yoga : from counterculture to pop culture / Andrea R. Jain.
pages cm
Includes bibliographical references.
ISBN 978-0-19-939024-3 (pbk. : alk. paper)—ISBN 978-0-19-939023-6
(cloth : alk. paper)   1. Yoga—Economic aspects.   2. Popular culture.   I. Title.
BL1238.52.J35 2014
181'.45—dc23
2014017038

For the loves of my life:

Tim Lyons—my companion, co-creator, and comrade and
Huxley Jain Lyons—my child and pure joy

Orthodoxy is the diehard of the world of thought.
It learns not, neither can it forget.

—ALDOUS HUXLEY

Contents

Preface

> There is therefore no central something to which the
> peripheral people were peripheral. One person's center is
> another's periphery.
> —WENDY DONIGER, *The Hindus* (2009: 29)

MY FIRST ENCOUNTER with a yoga guru occurred on July 1, 2006, in Rajasthan, India. It was quite literally face to face with Acharya Shri Mahaprajna (1920–2010), the *acharya* or monastic leader and guru of the Jain Shvetambara Terapanth.[1] Mahaprajna prescribed what he called *preksha dhyana*, literally "concentration of perception" but most often translated by insiders to the tradition as "insight meditation and yoga." One component of preksha dhyana is modern postural yoga, which includes a variety of regimens consisting of some combination of *asana* or "posture" synchronized with the breath through *pranayama* or "breath control."[2] In preksha dhyana, postural yoga is one component of a complex yoga system, which also includes meditation and relaxation techniques.

Of course, I had encountered postural yoga before this meeting, having lived in American cosmopolitan environments during childhood, college, and graduate school and thus having seen postural yoga practically everywhere I turned, from strip-mall yoga studios to advertisements for the Gap. I had even attended a semester-long postural yoga class while I was in college and continued to incorporate some of the practices I learned there into my daily exercise regimen. But this encounter with Mahaprajna and his preksha dhyana was particularly enlightening as it forced me, for the first time, to critically examine postural yoga as a transnational cultural product. Due to industrialization and the dominant and global socioeconomic forces of market capitalism, developments in the construction and practice of cultural products such as yoga have simultaneously occurred in urban areas across the globe. The stories of yoga in South

Asia, Europe, North America, the Middle East, and other regions of the world, therefore, are each a part of a larger global narrative.

I had just arrived in the city of Ladnun in the Marvar district of Rajasthan and was adjusting to its fiercely ascetic landscape. Ladnun is in the desert. It was the middle of the summer, and the temperature was well over a hundred degrees Fahrenheit. The sand was in my hair, clothes, and lungs. I could even feel it crunch between my teeth. This was my first meeting with Mahaprajna. I entered a largely empty room in which five or six *munis* sat quietly in front of a short table on which Mahaprajna sat elevated about a foot above the ground.[3] The Jain *acharya* was an elderly man, with a bald head and bare feet. He wore nothing but a white robe and a *muhpatti* or "mouth-shield."[4]

After explicating his view on what it means to self-identify as "Jain," he turned to me and asked if I was a "Jain," to which I replied, "No." He then asked, "Why wouldn't you want to be a Jain?" Although today we often rely on such distinguishing categories as *Jain* and *Hindu* to talk about what are perceived as identifiable, bounded South Asian religions, those terms have been far more fluid and contested in their applications throughout the history of religions. Yet it would be correct to state that the category *Jain* in at least most cases has been useful for identifying those individuals and institutions over the past twenty-five hundred years or so primarily in South Asia who have shared a certain dualist assessment of the world, which was tied to a particular understanding of history, and resulted in the construction of a particularly ascetic path toward salvation. Yet for Mahaprajna, I did not need to state my position on such matters in order to self-identify as Jain. In his encounter with an American scholar of religions, Mahaprajna was more concerned with defining Jain identity in terms of a desire for "universal peace and health" rather than in terms of membership in a particular religio-philosophical or social group committed to a shared ontology (system of ideas with regard to being or what *is*), history, and axiology (system of values or goals). Why, Mahaprajna was asking me, would anyone not want what he was so confident was the right path to "peace" and "health"?

Much of what being Jain was about, according to Mahaprajna, was yoga and, more specifically, yoga as a means to a modern conception of health and well-being. Furthermore, his vision of yoga intersected with much of what I tended to associate with the postural yoga market. I was surprised to witness such a position in someone who was a Jain monastic and thus embodied the very ascetic ideal that results from a characteristically

Jain worldview and practice. Mahaprajna's position on the importance of a modern conception of physical health and the means to get there posed the question of whether or not he represented a change in attitude toward the body from the traditional Jain denunciatory one, which perceives the body as something to be "conquered," as an obstacle to salvation.

In my study of South Asian religions, I had always been interested in the shifting nature of religion in its multifarious orientations toward the human body. In my encounters with different religio-somatic phenomena, I had consistently found myself asking: How is this idea about the body or body practice indicative of acclimation to shifting social contexts? I had been particularly interested in these questions with regard to the historical and contemporary structures and social implications of ascetic religious orientations toward the body. Consequently, in this encounter with Mahaprajna, I immediately asked whether or not the contrast between the traditional Jain attitude toward the body and that of this living Jain yoga guru reflected adaptations to his contemporary social context.

I could not grasp, and thus was set on a trajectory that would involve many years of research, the contrast between the world-, society-, and body-negating ascetic ideology of traditional Jain monastic thought and the active concern with modern conceptions of universal peace, physical health, and psychological well-being of Mahaprajna and his many disciples. Upon my return home from Rajasthan to Houston, Texas, I immediately began exploring the Terapanth center in my own city, where two *samanis*, female monastic disciples of Mahaprajna, lived and taught preksha dhyana. There I found an even greater contrast between what I understood as the Jain ascetic ideal of the Terapanth and what the samanis taught to mostly members of the South Asian Jain diaspora.[5]

I quickly accepted that indeed the phenomena I witnessed between Mahaprajna in Rajasthan and the samanis in Houston were transnational in scope. In their propagation of preksha dhyana, I was certain I was witnessing an attempt to establish continuity with a global market in which popularized varieties of postural yoga reflected dominant demands and needs. In other words, Mahaprajna and the samanis attempted to attract people to preksha dhyana by making it intersect with the global yoga market in which yoga served to fulfill aims specific to the context of a transnational consumer culture.

Individuals in India, the United States, and other parts of the world where postural yoga was becoming increasingly popular were undergoing shared cultural processes. The common trope that the popularization of yoga in the contemporary world reflects the transplantation of a cultural ware from "the East" to "the West" does not take into account that people of all regions and nations today are intertwined in many of the same cultural processes (see, e.g., Caldwell 2001: 25; Bryant and Ekstrand 2004; Williamson 2005: 149; and Williamson 2010). It is, therefore, unreasonable to retain the opposition of East and West or a notion of a static, isolated Indian culture, American culture, or otherwise.

I sought to explain how the symbols, practices, values, and ideas I encountered in the contemporary Terapanth relate to contemporary transnational cultural circumstances. How are members of the Terapanth invoking transnational social symbols and discourses? Mahaprajna's yoga betrayed many of the qualities of popularized varieties of postural yoga. For example, he appropriated modern scientific discourse and modern fitness methods hardly present in Jain traditions prior to the twentieth century, and he translated explanations of traditional Jain cultural symbols oriented around ascetic purification, such as fasting and vegetarianism, into modern biomedical terminology. Preksha dhyana, therefore, struck me as an attempt to resolve the tension between the ascetic disassociation from the body, society, and world, a commitment characteristic of Jain soteriology, and the popular needs and demands that fueled the global postural yoga market in the late twentieth and early twenty-first centuries.

To understand preksha dhyana's relationship to the global postural yoga market, I had to move beyond a face-to-face encounter with the Terapanth acharya and his immediate community and go from place to place in a methodological approach George Marcus terms *multi-sited ethnography* (Marcus 1995: 95–117). Marcus suggests, "[E]thnography is predicated upon attention to the everyday, an intimate knowledge of face-to-face communities and groups" (Marcus 1995: 99). For preksha dhyana to be ethnographically accounted for, I could not limit myself to a face-to-face encounter with a single site or even two sites. Mahaprajna, after all, prescribed his path toward peace and health for all human beings and thus sent the samanis throughout the world to disseminate his rendition of Jain thought and practice. The samanis sought to "take Jainism beyond the Jains" by means of the popular dissemination of preksha dhyana. They dispersed to numerous locations with the mission to diffuse that system to the greatest extent possible.

Since preksha dhyana intersects at so many points with postural yoga, I found myself trying to account for postural yoga's popularization in urban areas across the world. As I broadened the scope of my study to include postural yoga generally, the study increasingly required an ethnography of multiple sites. A multi-sited ethnography, as elegantly articulated by Marcus, "moves out from the single sites and local situations of conventional ethnographic research designs to examine the circulation of cultural meanings, objects, and identities in diffuse time-space" (Marcus 1995: 96). Such a methodological approach, according to Marcus, is a response to empirical changes in the world that result in the shifting locations of cultural production (Marcus 1995: 97). The empirical changes in the world I observe and analyze in the present study have occurred in the modern period and have involved processes of market capitalism, industrialization, globalization, and transnationalism, which have facilitated the increasing growth and spread of consumer culture. This study is concerned with a cultural object, postural yoga, that I argue is today largely a product of consumer culture. The construction, dissemination, and practice of postural yoga are the key dimensions for connecting multiple sites.

Marcus suggests that a certain assumption underlies the multi-sited ethnographic method: An ethnography of any single cultural formation in the world system is an ethnography of the system itself because it is the cultural formation produced across time and space that is the object of study (Marcus 1995: 99). In my analysis of postural yoga, therefore, I hope to not only better understand postural yoga, but also to better understand the transnational system within which it exists and thrives—that is, contemporary consumer culture.

From Ladnun and Houston, I set out to follow postural yoga through a series of associations and relationships to physical sites in London and throughout the United States and India. I followed it farther, through websites and publications, to other contemporary areas of cultural production. Contemporary popular culture defies the ability to locate any cultural object at one site or even several sites. And in the case of postural yoga, we cannot locate it in my chosen sites alone. However, as a practical move, this study uses them as windows into the incalculable sites of the construction, dissemination, and practice of postural yoga.

Finally, as argued by Marcus, multi-sited ethnography is "comparative...as a function of the fractured, discontinuous plane of movement and discovery among sites" (Marcus 1995: 102). Comparison, therefore, as a method is vital to my analysis, which seeks to understand postural yoga in its heterogeneous forms and locations. I evaluate, compare, and explore the relationships between various postural yoga systems and figures, attending not just to similarities across time and space but also, and especially, to discrepancies and incongruities. As I will suggest, the most important lesson from the history of yoga is that yoga is contextual and malleable. And the construction and practice of postural yoga alone are heterogeneous, perpetually shifting as one moves from one site to another. In other words, the same rule Wendy Doniger notes with regard to what is commonly termed *Hinduism*—"One person's center is another's periphery" (2009: 29)—applies to the world of postural yoga.

Self-Reflexivity and Heterogeneity in Contemporary Culture

Before embarking upon my study of postural yoga, I would like to provide some self-reflexive thoughts on the unique circumstances of my encounter with my subject. Questions with regard to the heterogeneity of cultural products are salient for the current study, which evaluates the ever-changing forms of yoga in the contemporary context of consumer culture, but also for me personally. After all, like postural yoga, I am a product of such heterogeneity and the consequent encounters between previously isolated cultural formations in the late twentieth century. I am the daughter of a white mother who grew up in a small blue-collar Protestant community in Illinois and an Indian father from Mumbai who was raised in an elite Jain Digambara family.[6]

Although my familial background did not determine my area of research—not consciously anyway—it did frequently come up in my ethnographic encounters simply as a consequence of my last name, which is "Jain." My consistent attempt to assert myself as "Jain...but not Jain" in the sense of name but not religious self-identity stirred interesting responses from my subjects that relate directly to questions regarding contemporary phenomena as products of encounters across what was previously non- (or at least rarely) traversable space.

When my Jain subjects were aware of my name, I was frequently reminded that my Jain identity was not something they were willing to compromise on given their commitments to a traditional Jain ontology that maintains karmic explanations for one's current state in the world. In other words, they were not willing to give up their karmic explanations of my Jain-ness. For them, I was not a product of my social context.

I was a Jain because my karma determined it be so. And my persistent attempts to assert my "Jain...but not Jain" identity just amused them— that is, they were unwilling to grant me agency in identifying as either "Jain" or "not Jain."

On the one hand, I found that, given my "Jain" status, my Jain subjects often expected that I would differentiate, in their favor of course, the "true" Jain tradition from "false" corruptions and likewise the "true" yoga tradition from "false" corruptions. For Jain and yoga traditions have a long history, much like religious individuals and institutions generally, of battling over authenticity. In the history of religions, orthodox representatives often frame change as part of reformation, a return to origins and authenticity rather than as appropriation or adaptation. Representatives maintain that reformations introduce qualities lost at some point that are now being rediscovered. Accordingly, they consider reformations in line with an eternal orthodoxy and see them as "purified" from heterodoxy, which corrupted original, authentic teachings over time.[7] My academic colleagues and friends, on the other hand, often looked to me to reduce my subjects', Jain or otherwise, concerns with yoga and health to *mere* socioeconomic and cultural adaptations, to mere commodifications or "borrowings."

As shocking as the Terapanth innovations are, however, I suggest that they do not deauthenticate it as a Jain tradition, but contribute to the stability of that particular institution in its present-day social context. Likewise, the innovations unique to postural yoga more broadly do not deauthenticate it as "true" or "authentic" yoga simply because they represent products of consumer culture. Postural yoga is a transnational product of yoga's encounter with global processes, particularly the rise and dominance of market capitalism, industrialization, globalization, and the consequent diffusion of consumer culture. To refer to its innovations as "cosmetic" or "borrowings," however, would undermine the ontological, axiological, narrative, and ritual functions and meanings of postural yoga for the practitioners I engage with in my study, the insiders to postural yoga.

If it could be conclusively shown that pop culture yoga was in part a result of the interaction between consumer ideology and values and yoga in the twentieth century, should any person seriously argue on that basis that it should therefore be dismissed from any notion of "true" or "authentic" yoga or reduced to mere borrowings? I suggest that it should not be dismissed and am inspired by John Cort's assertions in response to the reduction of Jain *bhakti* or "devotional" traditions to mere borrowings from Hinduism:

> At one level the issue of "borrowing" is really a nonissue. When a scholar argues that because a practice, institution, or belief has been borrowed from another tradition its role in the borrowing tradition is therefore of negligible importance, the scholar is making a fundamental error of judging the data by standards inappropriate to any form of objective scholarship. (Cort 2002: 60)

In the popular imagination and in much scholarship, postural yoga often is dismissed from any serious consideration of what yoga *is*. Some individuals and institutions, discussed in detail in proceeding chapters, have implicitly and explicitly criticized postural yoga as illegitimate or a corruption of the center of true yoga. But their portraits of postural yoga are misleading. In this study, I analyze how yoga has been perpetually context-sensitive, so there is no "legitimate," "authentic," "true," or "original" tradition, only contextualized ideas and practices organized around the term *yoga*. Postural yoga, then, should not be set apart as a mere accretion simply for its context sensitivity for the same reason I should not be judged as not *really* a person of color or not *really* a person of white Midwestern American heritage because my parents' relationship was possible only as a result of recent social circumstances.

Rather, if the popularization of postural yoga can be accounted for satisfactorily with recourse to explanations of yoga proponents responding to contemporary consumer cultural values, processes, and ideas, then our understanding of yoga itself needs to be modified, our understanding of the role of social context in the development of yoga as a whole needs to be modified, and our understanding of contemporary culture needs to be expanded.

Issues regarding borrowings and derivations are not reasons to disregard postural yoga but are important for helping us understand the history of yoga. The case of postural yoga evidences that the history of yoga includes processes of assimilation, commodification, branding, and consumption. This all encourages an expansion and reconceptualization of our understanding of yoga. If scholars of yoga study as equally meaningful all those ideas and practices that insiders to yoga systems over the centuries have called *yoga*, they find that yoga is a complex, heterogeneous cultural product, which is understood and practiced differently in different times and places, including contemporary consumer culture. Likewise, yoga more broadly is not one single thing. It is many things, and a significant part of the study of yoga generally and postural yoga in particular is the study of the strident disagreements over what yoga is, how it is to be practiced, and by whom.

It is, therefore, neither within my capacity nor within my interests to delineate the boundaries of a true, authentic, or original yoga tradition. In response to the scholarly tendency to write off Jain bhakti traditions as mere borrowings from Hindu bhakti, Cort rejected all questions of legitimacy, instead arguing that, in his sociohistorical analysis, "the legitimacy of Jain bhakti is not a subject that is open to scholarly debate" (Cort 2002: 60). Likewise, the legitimacy of preksha dhyana, Bikram Yoga, Anusara Yoga, or Iyengar Yoga, among other varieties of postural yoga, is not a subject to debate in the current study.

As postural yoga becomes increasingly a part of pop culture around the world, it is more often subject to complex interactions between not only local private and public individuals and institutions, but also transnational corporations and state governments. Postural yoga is a valuable commodity available for exchange through globally franchised corporations, such as the Bikram's Yoga College of India and Anusara, Inc. With each exchange, postural yoga morphs into new forms. Increasingly, individual yoga proponents and opponents, transnational corporations, and state governments attempt to locate a center to yoga in their arguments both for and against intellectual copyright, patent, and trademark claims on yoga products and services. Many individuals and corporations have, often in an effort to control the fiercely profitable yoga market, registered thousands of intellectual property claims on yoga products and services, while state governments have attempted to enforce regulatory laws on the yoga market. Some Hindu and scholarly antipostural yoga movements and thinkers have reacted to the profitable yoga market by attempting to exercise power over defining what counts as true, authentic yoga and what amounts to mere commodification or corruption.

The purpose of the current study is not to establish what counts as true, authentic yoga or determine who rightfully owns yoga. The purpose is, rather, multifaceted and includes the following: to provide a major chapter in the history of modern yoga by attending to the question of what cultural changes enabled postural yoga to become a part of pop culture; to demonstrate that popularized postural yoga systems are not mere "commodifications" or "borrowings" but idiosyncratic and complex creations all of which insiders call *yoga*—in other words, even in consumer culture, yoga is in part what yogis say it is; and to bring critical scrutiny to bear on social and religious expressions in popularized yoga systems.

In my discussion of yoga and, more specifically, modern yoga I want to avoid implying that a monolithic tradition exists. Although in popular and academic discourse, we abstractly speak about *yoga* in the singular, there is, in reality, no single yoga, only *yogas*. I use the singular term *yoga* throughout this study because this is the term privileged today by those who "do yoga" as it is colloquially put. I deliberately avoid reifying yoga as something that has an essence or core, however, by not capitalizing it and by illuminating, wherever possible, the divergences and differences between yoga systems.[8]

In an attempt to speak to a wider audience that includes the variety of contemporary people who do yoga, rather than simply that of my academic peers, I deliberately approach the study of postural yoga through a more accessible style than traditional academic studies. This book seeks to raise a series of questions that speak to wider cultural concerns and constituencies than are usually appealed to in academia. I hope to speak to many audiences about why so many consumers across the world, including many who I hope will read this book, are choosing yoga as a part of their everyday regimens. I also hope to speak about why some consumers reject it outright, sometimes with great hostility.

Yoga undergoes certain acts of assimilation to its current social context. However, as convincingly argued by Max Weber, religion is a process of assimilation to the contingencies of social life. Likewise is yoga. I thus remain neutral and make no attempts to locate what is "authentic" or "original" in the world of yoga or, more specifically, postural yoga. And I take its many expressions seriously as complex social phenomena. My interest and capacity as a scholar are to convincingly argue that postural yoga, like religion, is nonstable, ever-adaptive, and never monolithic. One postural yogi's center is another's periphery.

Acknowledgments

OVER THE LAST several years as I worked on this project, I have had the privilege and pleasure of meeting and exchanging ideas with many wonderful people. I must first thank Jeffrey J. Kripal. Jeff was my graduate school supervisor. He has also been a constant source of mentorship, friendship, insight, humor, and support. In the difficult moments, I have leaned on his unwavering confidence in me. I deeply admire and appreciate him.

Many others played significant roles in my research and thinking. The following individuals deserve special mention. I am indebted to my former professors and now friends, G. William Barnard and Mark A. Chancey, for challenging me when I needed it most during my undergraduate career at Southern Methodist University and for their unending inspiration, moral support, and encouragement. As I worked through the early stages of the current project during my graduate career at Rice University, the critiques and guidance I received from, not only Jeff, but also James D. Faubion and William B. Parsons proved to be invaluable. I am also grateful for the following friends and colleagues at Indiana University-Purdue University Indianapolis who graciously read and offered feedback on rough sketches of chapters or provided ongoing advice and encouragement: David M. Craig, Edward E. Curtis, Philip Goff, Timothy D. Lyons, Peter J. Thuesen, and John J. Tilley. I received additional guidance, friendship, and support from my peers and mentors in the 2011–2012 Teaching and Learning Workshop for Pre-Tenure Asian and Asian American Religion and Theology Faculty. I am especially indebted to Zayn Kassam for her ongoing mentorship and friendship. Among the others who offered comments and critiques that significantly enhanced the current project are Joseph S. Alter, Christopher Key Chapple, Ellen Goldberg, Amy Hollywood, Stuart R. Sarbacker, and Mark Singleton.

The following institutions generously supported various stages of my writing, travel, and research: the Department of Religious Studies, the School of Humanities, and the Office of Fellowships and Undergraduate Research at Rice University; the Andrew W. Mellon Foundation; the International Summer School for Jain Studies; the Jain Vishva Bharati Institute; the Wabash Center for Teaching and Learning in Theology and Religion; and the Department of Religious Studies and the School of Liberal Arts at Indiana University-Purdue University Indianapolis.

I would like to thank my editor at Oxford University Press, Cynthia Read. Cynthia demonstrated patience and support while I completed my book. She encouraged my early, at times undeveloped, thoughts and a book proposal that needed to be reworked several times. I am also appreciative of the anonymous readers for Oxford University Press who provided extensive comments and suggestions. Their close readings of the first draft of the manuscript and my consideration of their careful responses greatly enhanced the final product.

Some parts of this book have appeared in different incarnations elsewhere—for instance, in essays published in *Religion Dispatches* and *Himal Southasian*. Part of Chapter Three appeared in a different form in "The Dual-Ideal of the Ascetic and Healthy Body: The Jain Terāpanth and Modern Yoga in the Context of Late Capitalism," *Nova Religio* 15(3) (February 2012): 29–50. Parts of Chapters Three and Four appeared in different forms in "Branding Yoga: The Cases of Iyengar Yoga, Siddha Yoga, and Anusara Yoga," *Approaching Religion* 2/2: 3–17 (2012); and in "Muktananda: Entrepreneurial Godman, Tantric Hero," in *Gurus of Modern Yoga*, edited by Mark Singleton and Ellen Goldberg (New York: Oxford University Press, 2013). Parts of Chapter Six appeared in a different form in "The Malleability of Yoga: A Response to Christian and Hindu Opponents of the Popularization of Yoga," *Journal of Hindu-Christian Studies* 25 (2012): 3–10. An earlier version of Chapter Six appeared as "Who Is to Say Modern Yoga Practitioners Have It All Wrong? On Hindu Origins and Yogaphobia," *Journal of the American Academy of Religion* 82(2) (June 2014): 427–471.

Note on Transliteration

HINDI, SANSKRIT, AND other non-English language terms are italicized upon their first usage with the exception of terms that have become a part of the English language lexicon, such as "guru" and "yoga." Transliteration does not employ diacritical marks and follows the custom of the particular movement under consideration whenever relevant. Terms that sometimes appear together, such as *yogasutras*, are rendered separated (*Yoga Sutras*) to aid a general audience.

Selling Yoga

I

Premodern Yoga Systems

*"Yoga" has a wider range of meanings than nearly any
other word in the entire Sanskrit lexicon.*
—DAVID GORDON WHITE (2012: 2)

WHEN WE THINK of yoga today, most of us envision spandex-clad, perspiring, toned bodies brought together in a room filled with yoga mats and engaged in a fitness ritual set apart from day-to-day life.[1] In that space, Christians, Hindus, atheists, and others gather to enhance something they deem sacred: their bodies, their selves.[2] In popularized yoga classes today, we most frequently find some variety of postural yoga, a fitness regimen made up of sequences of often onerous *asanas* or bodily postures, the movement through which is synchronized with the breath by means of *pranayama* or "breath control."

Though these are images never seen before in the history of yoga, well-known proponents and opponents alike associate them with the "ancient yoga" of South Asia, claiming it is there that we can locate this widespread practice's "origins."[3] In popular yoga discourse, claims to a linear trajectory of transmission—premodern yoga functions as what Mark Singleton describes as "the touchstone of authenticity" for proponents of modern yoga (Singleton 2010: 14)—are frequently made and assumed to be historically accurate. For example, postural yoga giants B. K. S. Iyengar (b. 1918) and K. Pattabhi Jois (1915–2009) have claimed direct historical ties between their postural yoga methods and ancient yoga traditions. While Iyengar has historically claimed ties between Iyengar Yoga and the ancient yoga transmission going at least as far back as the *Yoga Sutras* (circa 350–450 C.E.), he recently introduced a Sanskrit invocation to Patanjali at the beginning of each Iyengar Yoga class in order to further associate his yoga system with that transmission.[4] In like manner, Jois has suggested that verses from the earliest Vedas delineate the nine postures of the *suryanamaskar* sequences of postures in his Ashtanga Vinyasa yoga system (Singleton 2010: 221–222, n. 4).[5]

In the popular imagination, the development of a monolithic yoga tradition can be traced back to the *Yoga Sutras*, the ancient doctrines of the earliest Vedas (circa 1700–1500 B.C.E.), or to even more ancient origins over 5,000 years ago in the Indus Valley Civilization (circa 2500–1500 B.C.E.).[6] Consider, for example, a statement about yoga on a PBS website featuring a special series entitled *The Story of India*:

> Seals from the Indus Valley Civilization dating to the 3rd millennium BCE depict what appear to be yogic poses. The *Bhagavad Gita, Puranas,* and *Mahabharata* are among the texts that describe yoga's teachings, which were codified at about 150 BCE in the *Yoga Sutra* written by Patanjali. (PBS 2008)

Such statements about the history of yoga, which presume an unbroken lineage, do not reflect historical reality, which is far more complex and about which scholars are far more uncertain, especially given the extreme ambiguities involved in dating South Asian texts, events, and figures.

Yet, because such statements are common in popular discourse and make up the narratives that function to reinforce the postural yoga world's self-images, values, ideas, and practices, any study of postural yoga necessitates serious consideration of yoga's actual premodern history. For that reason, this chapter provides the premodern backdrop for the modern popularization of postural yoga. Though there is not nearly enough room in this chapter to provide exhaustive coverage of what scholars have uncovered about premodern yoga, I draw on recent secondary scholarship in order to make two points particularly relevant to my analysis of the popularization of yoga. First, modern postural yoga is radically distinct from premodern yoga traditions. Second, premodern yoga traditions were not monolithic; rather, they were dramatically heterogeneous, taking a wide range of forms, including Hindu, Buddhist, and Jain ones. I hope to frame these points in nuanced ways that challenge common assumptions about the history of yoga, especially the assumption that a static, monolithic yoga tradition gradually, increasingly, and in a linear way underwent popularization from the nineteenth to the late twentieth centuries.

We will look at the modern history and recent popularization of yoga much more closely in proceeding chapters where I will suggest, on the one hand, that the early history of modern yoga features yoga systems that are distinct from premodern ones and reflect instead modern countercultural ideas and values.[7] I will add that popularized systems of modern yoga, on the other hand, are also distinct from premodern ones but instead reflect modern consumer cultural ideas and values.[8] For now, it is sufficient to note that there is no direct, unbroken lineage between the South Asian premodern yoga systems and modern postural yoga (Alter 2004; de Michelis 2004; Singleton 2010). In other words, today's popularized yoga systems are new, not continuations of some static premodern yoga tradition from which practitioners and nonpractitioners alike often claim they originate. Even postures and breathing exercises were marginal to the most widely cited sources on yoga prior to the twentieth century, and the forms of postures and breathing exercises that were present in those sources dramatically differ from those idiosyncratic forms found in postural yoga today (Singleton 2010). For example, though pranayama appears in both the *Bhagavad Gita* and the *Yoga Sutras*, it means the "complete cessation of breathing" in those sources (Bronkhorst 2007: 26–27) rather than the synchronization of breath with postural movement found in most postural yoga sites today.[9] Furthermore, the dominant aims of postural yoga—health, stress reduction, beauty, and overall well-being according to modern biomedicine and contemporary cultural standards (Alter 2004; de Michelis 2004; Strauss 2005; Newcombe 2007; Singleton 2010)—are also absent in those sources. These absences even apply to the most widely cited "classical" sources on yoga, including the *Yoga Sutras*, the *Bhagavad Gita* and other material from the *Mahabharata*, as well as the *Yoga Upanishads*.

Since Mircea Eliade's distinguished monograph *Yoga: Immortality and Freedom* (1990 [1958]), a late Orientalist study concerned with identifying the "ideal of Yoga" across traditions (363), many scholars have preferred to attend to the particularities of yoga traditions, which vary based largely on social context. These scholars have produced studies that resist Orientalist misrepresentations of yoga as having a single "ideal." In other words, they reject any notion of yoga as timeless, monolithic, and characterized by an unchanging essence, instead suggesting that empirical data evidence that premodern yoga systems, made up of a variety of complex ritual, religious, philosophical, and narrative traditions, never appear outside of social contexts. By drawing on a number of such studies, I will emphasize premodern yoga's context-sensitivity, heterogeneity, and malleability, rather than any central quality or essence presumed by some to be present across systems.

Based on historical scholarship that confirms that premodern yoga took a wide variety of forms, Geoffrey Samuel defines it broadly and heterogeneously as composed of "disciplined and systematic techniques for the training and control of the human mind-body complex, which are also understood as techniques for the reshaping of human consciousness towards some kind of higher goal" (Samuel 2008: 2). Samuel argues for a "culturally and historically situated understanding," since yoga continuously undergoes transformations in response to shifting temporal and spatial contexts (Samuel 2007: 186). He adds:

> [Yoga] has retained some of its integrity as a specific set of techniques for self-cultivation through all of these transformations. To make sense of such a historical complex and varied phenomenon as yoga, it is, however, essential to retain as much awareness as possible of the social environment and historical specificity of each specific context within which it was adopted and transformed. In this way, we can begin to give meaning to each of these various forms of yoga, and to understand them within the life and culture of those who created them and shaped them. (Samuel 2007: 186)

Evidence of the existence of yoga has been claimed to go as far back as the Indus Valley Civilization, which can be dated to circa 2500 to 1500 B.C.E. Others claim such evidence goes as far back as the earliest known collection of Hindu literature, the Vedas, the first of which can be dated to circa 1700 to 1500 B.C.E. Contemporary scholars debate whether or not archaeological artifacts from the Indus Valley Civilization or textual evidence from the early Vedas are evidence of yoga's origins and resist treating any single textual source on yoga as the yoga "ur-text."

Those in favor of the argument that yoga was present in the Indus Valley Civilization point to specific artifacts, especially the famously titled "Pashupati Seal" (Mohenjo-daro seal No. 420), which depicts a possibly ithyphallic figure with horns, surrounded by animals, and in what some interpret to be a seated yoga posture.[10] The seal was named after what Sir John Marshall, Director General of the Archaeological

Survey of India, thought was the figure's resemblance to the Hindu deity Shiva (Marshall 1931: 7). Shiva is nicknamed Pashupati or "Lord of the Beasts," and Hindu devotees celebrate him for his outstanding yogic abilities. Thomas McEvilley points to other Indus Valley seals and suggests they depict early forms of postures found in much later yoga systems, including modern postural yoga, specifically the *utkata asana* (*Gheranda Samhita* II.27) or *mulabandha asana* (Iyengar 1966: Fig. 459–463) (McEvilley 1981: 49).

The links between the Indus Valley Civilization and yoga, however, are highly speculative. Doris Srinivasan (1984) reviews the artifacts cited for the existence of proto-Shiva forms—most significantly certain characteristics of the Pashupati Seal[11]—and concludes that there is nothing that conclusively shows that the seal depicts a proto-Shiva figure. Samuel adds that any evidence of yoga in the Indus Valley Civilization is "so dependent on reading later practices into the material that it is of little or no use for constructing any kind of history of practices" (2008: 8).

Since interpreting material culture poses a number of difficulties for the modern historian of yoga, our knowledge of premodern yoga primarily depends on the historical-critical study of the South Asian literary tradition. This is the case even though locally constituted yoga traditions were probably distinct from textual ones (Smith, Frederick 2011), and texts do not tell us exactly how yoga was put into practice (Samuel 2011: 311). Despite such complications, textual traditions reveal much about the multifarious nature of premodern yoga.

The term *yoga* in the South Asian literary tradition had a wide range of meanings specific to particular contexts. In fact, according to David Gordon White:

> "Yoga" has a wider range of meanings than nearly any other word in the entire Sanskrit lexicon. The act of yoking an animal, as well as the yoke itself, is called yoga. In astronomy, a conjunction of planets or stars, as well as a constellation, is called yoga. When one mixes together various substances, that, too, can be called yoga. The word yoga has also been employed to denote a device, a recipe, a method, a strategy, a charm, an incantation, fraud, a trick, an endeavor, a combination, union, an arrangement, zeal, care, diligence, industriousness, discipline, use, application, contact, a sum total, and the Work of alchemists. But this is by no means an exhaustive list. (White 2012: 2)

The term *yoga* makes an appearance in South Asian literature's earliest known text, the *Rig Veda Samhita* (circa fifteenth century B.C.E.). Samuel suggests, however, "There is nothing [in the Rigveda or Atharvaveda]...to imply yogic practice, in the sense of a developed set of techniques for operating with the mind-body complex" (2008: 8). Rather, the term *yoga* (from the Sanskrit root *yuj*, meaning "to bind" or "to yoke") refers to the yoke used to bind an animal to a plow or chariot and also to an entire war chariot (White 2012: 3). More broadly, yoga refers to wartime itself (White 2012: 3). Vedic hymns also refer to the gods moving about heaven and earth on yogas as well as priests yoking themselves "to poetic inspiration and so journeying—if only with the mind's eye or cognitive apparatus—across the metaphorical distance that separated the world of the gods from the words of their hymns" (White 2012: 4). Yoga's warrior connotation was prevalent in ancient India as evidenced by the later text, the *Mahabharata* (circa 200 B.C.E. to 400 C.E.), in which dying heroic warriors are described as *yoga-yukta*, "yoked to yoga," the chariot believed to deliver them to heaven (White 2009: 73). White explains:

> The image of the dying warrior who is "hitched to his rig" [*yoga-yukta*], or "ready to hitch up" in order to advance upward to the highest path, formed the basis for the earliest yoga paradigm, which privileged a dynamic of outward movement and conquest. Only later, in the period of the latest strata of the epics and of the "classical" Upaniṣads (i.e., the third to fourth centuries CE) would the goal of yogic practice be transferred to a place hidden within the body's deepest recesses, and the seven solar winds internalized into the inner breaths. Yet, even after this inward turn has taken place, the yoga of the chariot warrior persists in the language of later visionary practice. (White 2009: 73)

In the sense of a systematic set of techniques, Samuel and Johannes Bronkhorst both suggest that yoga developed in the context of a non-Vedic religious culture, the *shramana* culture of "Greater Magadha" (Bronkhorst 2007: 1–9), also known as the "Central Gangetic region" (Samuel 2008: 8). The shramana culture was primarily composed of Buddhist, Jain, and Ajivika renouncers (circa the sixth and fifth centuries B.C.E.), those who rejected Brahmanical orthodoxy and whose axiological focus was salvation from the conventional and ordinary world, a goal that required ascetic practices.

Though participants in the early Brahmanical culture referred to their own ascetic techniques as *tapas*, they referred to the ascetic techniques found in the shramana culture as *yoga* (Bronkhorst 2011: 318–321).[12] In fact, *yoga* was first used as a term for a systematic set of ascetic techniques in Brahmanical sources but in reference to Buddhist practice (Bronkhorst 2011: 318).[13] Although some shramana and Brahmanical texts describe ascetic practices that are based on "some shared assumptions," those assumptions were not a part of the early Brahmanical tradition (Bronkhorst 2007: 28; Samuel 2008: 189).

Later, the shramana culture influenced the Brahmanical one (Bronkhorst 2007: 28), and consequently the Brahmanical emphasis on the ideal male warrior slowly transformed into the inner war of the *brahmacarin* or male celibate renouncer (Samuel 2008: 185).[14] This celibate role at first applied to the "semi-ascetic (but married) role of the Brahman within caste society" but, over a long time, came to include the "fully-ascetic role of the *saṃnyāsin* outside caste society proper" (Samuel 2008: 188).[15]

Though they differed from each other with regard to many aspects of belief and practice, the shramana traditions shared an assessment of rebirth as undesirable because of the preponderance of violence and suffering in the world. Consequently, they were organized around soteriological (salvation-oriented) goals, namely salvation from rebirth into the world. Bronkhorst suggests there were three main currents concerned with rebirth and karmic retribution and how to stop them (2007: 15–34). The Jain current was based on the assumption that abstention from all bodily and mental action prevents karmic retribution and thus rebirth. Buddhists prescribed a path concerned with controlling intention and, more specifically, requiring the cessation of desire. The third path, which was a product of the shramana culture but cannot be associated with any single particular movement within it (Bronkhorst 2007: 28), was based on the idea that knowledge of the nonactive nature of the self prevents karmic retribution and thus rebirth. Brahmanical orthodoxy slowly came to appropriate shramana ideas, especially from the last current. In fact, according to Bronkhorst:

> Knowledge of the self as requirement for attaining liberation became a potent force in classical Brahmanism, and is a fundamental ingredient of all the classical schools of Brahmanical philosophy, with the exception of Mīmāṃsā. (Bronkhorst 2007: 32)

Though some of the Brahmanical paths toward salvation required postures and breathing exercises, the most widely cited Brahmanical sources on soteriological systems of yoga emphasize meditative or devotional techniques. The *Katha Upanishad* (circa third century B.C.E.), for example, provides the first extant systematic account of yoga. Consider the following verses:

When the five organs of knowledge stand still together with the mind (*manas*), and the intellect (*buddhi*) does not stir, that they call the highest course (10). This they consider as Yoga, a firm fixing of the senses. Then one becomes careful, for Yoga is the origin and the end (11). (*Katha Upanishad* 6:10–11, quoted in Bronkhorst 2007: 25–26)

The author concludes by stating that "the whole method of Yoga" has been presented (*Katha Upanishad* 6:18, quoted in Bronkhorst 2007: 25–26). Yoga, according to this account, includes a number of characteristics that, in varying degrees, constituted some later yoga systems, including a yoga physiology; a nondualist ontology—*atman*, the individual self, is identical to *Brahman*, the cosmic essence; a hierarchy of mind–body constituents—the senses, the mind, the intellect, and so forth; the idea that the realization of higher states of consciousness requires an ascent through the mind–body constituents; and the use of mantras, acoustic spells or formulas (White 2012: 4).

Yoga also appears in the *Shvetashvatara Upanishad* (circa third century B.C.E.). The text directs the aspirant:

Holding the body straight, three parts of it stretched up, causing the senses to enter into the heart by means of the mind, the wise one should cross over all the frightening streams with the help of the raft which is Brahman (8). Having here suppressed his breaths and having brought his movements under control (*yukacesta*), when his breath has been diminished, he should take breath through his nose. Being careful, the wise one should restrain (*dhārayeta*) his mind like that chariot yoked with vicious horses (9). (*Shvetashvatara Upanishad* 2:8–9, quoted in Bronkhorst 2007: 26)

In this context, body practices are apparently central.

Yoga also makes an appearance in Brahmanical literature included in the category of *smriti* (that is, regarded as being of human authorship), which comprises texts concerned with *dharma* or rules of conduct and fantastic tales about powerful people and deities (the epics—the *Mahabharata* and the *Ramayana*—and the *Puranas*). Some authors attempt to fit what were initially ascetic ideas into Brahmanical themes, most notably dharma, the duties of high-caste male Hindus as determined by their *varna* or caste/social class and *ashrama* or stage of life (Olivelle 1993; Bronkhorst 2007). The householder life of most high-caste adult Hindus affirms the values of duty to society (dharma), wealth (*artha*), and erotic and aesthetic pleasure (*kama*). In short, the householder affirms worldly life and social values in pursuit of health, wealth, and, more generally, a better life in this lifetime and the next as well as general social stability through maintaining the strict rules of a hierarchical society. Ascetic ideas common to yoga traditions, however, were also incorporated into "the orbit of dharma":

> The *āśrama* system, it appears, sought to bring rival and often mutually exclusive life styles within the orbit of *dharma* by extending the use and meaning of *āśrama*. To call a mode of life an *āśrama*, therefore, was to give that life a theological meaning within the context of *dharma*.... The proponents of the system, in effect, were telling their Brāhmaṇical audience that the life of a celibate ascetic or student is as good as the life of a holy householder. (Olivelle 1993: 26)

Some sections of the *Mahabharata* (composed between circa 200 B.C.E. and 300 C.E.), for example, testify to the Brahmanical appropriation of yoga and the goal of *moksha* (Fitzgerald 2012: 44):

> [The "Prescription for *Yoga*:" Chapter 12.289 of the *Mahābhārata*] offers a glimpse of a well-developed tradition of reflection and praxis on body and mind that on its face is directed toward freeing a person in different ways—Absolute Liberation, *mokṣa*, and, by merging with the Supreme God Nārāyaṇa in the end, beatitude. At the same time, its *yoga*-harnessing can be, and is, directed toward the development of very high degrees of power and control within the phenomenal world for as long as the *yogin* may wish. And finally, this text presents all of this as a self-conscious "School" of thought (a *darśana*, a "View" of important matters of reality and knowledge) to be known as the "Yoga" School...(Fitzgerald 2012: 47)

The *Yoga Sutras*, most frequently ascribed to a figure by the name of Patanjali, includes 195 aphorisms on yoga, a discipline that also requires body practices. The *Yoga Sutras* are philosophically grounded in Samkhya dualism (Bronkhorst 1981; Larson 1989; Larson 1999; Larson 2012), which maintains that consciousness, *purusha*, is ontologically distinct from *prakriti*, materiality. *Prakriti* includes all aspects of material existence, from the body to ordinary awareness. The *Yoga Sutras* emphasize "meditation train-ing relating to the functioning of ordinary awareness (*citta-vṛtti*)" (Larson 2012: 73). Through meditation, the aspirant strives to achieve the "cessation of the functioning of ordinary awareness" (*citta-vṛtti-nirodha*) (*Yoga Sutras* 1.2), a yogic process that leads up to the key intuition that "ordinary aware-ness" is *kevala* or "isolated" from "consciousness" (Larson 2012: 78).

The yoga *sadhana* or "practice" that leads to this intuition is composed of eight "limbs." The first five limbs (*Yoga Sutras* 2:28–55) are "external limbs," which Gerald Larson defines as "largely practical, preparatory exercises" (Larson 2012: 79). These external limbs are (1) *yama*: behav-ioral restraints common in South Asian renouncer traditions—*ahimsa* (nonviolence), *satya* (telling the truth), *asteya* (restraint from stealing), *brahmacharya* (celibacy), and *aparigraha* (restraint from attachment); (2) *niyama*: ritual observances; (3) *asana*: postures; (4) *pranayama*: "breath control" exercises; and (5) *pratyahara*: "sense withdrawal" exercises. The final three limbs (*Yoga Sutras* 3:1–8), called "internal limbs," are described as "comprehensive reflection" (*samyama*) (Larson 2012: 80) and are (1) *dha-rana*: "spatial fixation on the object of meditation;" (2) *dhyana*: "temporal flow regarding the object of meditation;" and (3) *samadhi*: "cultivation of one-pointed 'concentration'" (Larson 2012: 78).

Although meditation is usually interpreted to be the preeminent com-ponent of yoga in the *Yoga Sutras*, numerous techniques, including tech-niques associated with contemporary postural yoga, namely asana and pranayama, are prerequisites for successful meditation. Asana, however, here includes "simply any posture of the body that is 'comfortably steady' for the sake of meditation practice ([*Yoga Sutras*] 2:46)" (Larson 2012: 80), and pranayama here entails "cutting off the movement of breathing out and breathing in" (*Yoga Sutras* 2:49, quoted in Bronkhorst 2007: 26–27), which serves to "increase the periods of the retention of breath (either after inhalation or exhalation)" (Larson 2012: 80; Larson cites *Yoga Sutras* 2:50). Therefore asana and pranayama in the *Yoga Sutras* do not resemble the types of asana and pranayama that dominate popularized varieties of postural yoga today.

According to the *Yoga Sutras*, the key method for attaining salvation is meditation whereby one realizes the self as pure consciousness, distinct from the mind–body complex. Similar, though not identical, systems appear in the late Upanishad, the *Maitrayaniya Upanishad*, which includes a six-fold yoga system, and in Virahanka Haribhadra's Jain text, the *Yoga Bindu* (circa 550 C.E.), which includes a five-fold yoga path (Williams 1965; Dixit 1968; Chapple 2003).

Turning inward and realizing that the self is pure consciousness was, however, not the only aim of early systematic yoga systems. Rather, turning outward, toward external objects or beings (a yogic process we tend to associate with later tantric yoga systems), was a common and perhaps the *most* common aim of early yoga systems. White, in fact, pushes against a vision of yoga as an inner-directed practice, based on a "closed" model of the body, and points out that yoga has often been about the body as "open" (White 2006: 6–12). According to White:

> This, I would argue is the most perennial and pervasive understanding of yoga in South Asia: not the identification of the individual self with the universal Self in meditative isolation (*kaivalyam*), but rather the yoking of the mind-body complex to an absolute located outside of the self—often behind the sun—or to that of other bodies, other selves ... (White 2006: 12)

Yoga was a term used in some sections of the *Mahabharata*, for example, to refer to a dying warrior's attempts to transfer himself to the sun (White 2006: 7–8). It was also used in the *Mahabharata* (White 2006: 8–10), as well as in Hemacandra's Jain text, the *Yoga Shastra*, to refer to techniques for transferring the practitioner's consciousness into another body (Qvarnström 2002). Even the *Yoga Sutras*, though usually interpreted as being concerned with meditative isolation (especially according to those who tend to reify a notion of "classical" yoga), refers to both of these applications of the term *yoga* (White 2006:10–11; see also Whicher 2002–2003).[16]

We will look at the reification of classical yoga more closely in proceeding chapters, but for now I would simply like to note that the concept is primarily a result of nineteenth-century Orientalist scholarship as well as Indian reform movements, most notably that of Swami Vivekananda (1863–1902), that prescribed a so-called classical form of yoga, usually termed *raja yoga* or "royal yoga." Although evidence does not suggest that the *Yoga Sutras* consistently functioned as the primary source on yoga in South Asia, it is frequently identified in popular discourse as the primary source or ur-text of what has become a reified concept of classical yoga—consider PBS's reference to the *Yoga Sutras* as *the* codification of yoga (PBS 2008).

The other frequently cited source on so-called classical yoga is the *Bhagavad Gita* (circa second century B.C.E. to first century C.E.). This text consists of a dialogue between the warrior, Arjuna, and his charioteer, Krishna, on the eve of a great war. The dialogue serves as a key scene from the *Mahabharata*. Krishna, who slowly reveals himself as Bhagavan, the transcendent Lord, prescribes yoga as a multivalent path to salvation through him. That path requires detachment from the fruits of actions (*karma yoga*), *bhakti* or "devotion" to Krishna (*bhakti yoga*), and the cultivation of mystical knowledge (*jnana yoga*).

The *Bhagavad Gita* and the *Yoga Sutras* are traditionally identified as Hindu texts. Yet the reification of the ideas and practices prescribed in those texts as exclusively Hindu is problematic. Buddhist and other non-Brahmanical renouncer traditions influenced the author of the *Yoga Sutras* (Bronkhorst 1993; Larson 1989). The *Yoga Sutras*, furthermore, require the practitioner to move beyond identifications of the self with notions tied to the mind–body complex, which, as interpreted by Edwin Bryant, would include any notion of religious identity (Bryant 2011). And yoga traditions based on the *Bhagavad Gita* state that individuals outside of the Brahmanical fold, and therefore outside of what is traditionally categorized as *Hindu*, can attain the highest states of devotion and therefore salvation (Bryant 2011).

An argument for an exclusively Hindu definition of yoga generally is problematic, since the history of yoga suggests that there was a "general climate of thought" in which participants drew from and reworked a shared set of religio-philosophical categories as well as textual traditions (Samuel 2008: 216). Examples include exchanges between the Buddhist Madhyamika school (second century C.E.), the Buddhist Yogacara school (third to fourth century C.E.), schools based on the *Yoga Sutras* (fourth to fifth century C.E.), Advaita Vedanta (circa eighth century C.E.), and Haribhadra Yakini-Putra's Jain *Yoga Drishti Samuccaya* (eighth century C.E.) (on exchanges between traditions, see, e.g., De la Vallée Poussin 1936–1937; Dixit 1968; Larson 1989; Bronkhorst 1993; Bronkhorst 1998; Chapple 2003; Qvarnström 2003: 131–133; Samuel 2008: 216–218, 232). For example, Haribhadra, in his *Yoga Drishti Samuccaya*, appears to have considerably drawn from the *Yoga Sutras*, Buddhist sources, as well as tantric sources in setting forth an eight-fold yoga path (Dixit 1968; Chapple 2003).

For all of these reasons, according to Samuel:

> [I]t is important to take 'yoga' in a wide sense, and to include the variety of related Buddhist and Jain practices, which may or may nor [*sic*] be called yoga, as well as the yogic and tantric traditions within the various religious currents that eventually led to modern Hinduism...developments within these various traditions were closely entwined with each other. (Samuel 2007: 179)

In Chapter Six, I will discuss in detail contemporary opponents of the popularization of yoga who define yoga as Hindu and will suggest that there is no historical precedence for such a narrow definition. For now, it is important to note that for many historical reasons, responsible historians avoid reifying the boundaries between South Asian yoga systems by ignoring the exchanges between participants in those systems.

In addition to avoiding the reification of boundaries between South Asian yoga systems, it is also important to avoid a reified notion of classical yoga since South Asian yoga persistently changed over time. Especially around the seventh and eighth centuries, yoga was reworked to a dramatic extent and came to include innovative ideas, largely with regard to the aim of immortality and a new interpretation of *prana*, the primary component of what was believed to be a subtle body (Samuel 2008: 255, 271–290).[17] The textual traditions found in the Buddhist and Hindu *Tantras* as well as Jain appropriations of tantra, for example, maintained much from earlier yoga systems but also introduced radical innovations (White 2012: 12).[18]

As a component of tantra, yoga served to increasingly refine consciousness, not as a means to salvation from embodied existence, but as a means to achieving a state of divine consciousness while remaining in embodied existence (White 2012: 12). In the *Tantras* alone, the term *yoga* has a wide range of meanings, including "practice" or "discipline" in a broad sense; the goal of yoga (that is, "conjunction," "union," or self-deification); an entire tantric soteriological system; in Buddhist *Tantras*, the dual sense of both the means and ends of practice; a program of meditation or visualization; or specific types of discipline (White 2012: 13).

Tantra came in both exoteric and esoteric forms. Exoteric practices included visualization, ritual sacrifice, devotion, and mantra as means to gradually achieving identification with the divine. Esoteric traditions combined the above practices with the idea that the practitioner could instantly and directly experience the divine but only by intentionally transgressing normative ethical and purity standards. Esoteric practices included the symbolic or real consumption of forbidden substances, such as semen and menstrual blood, and ritual sex with conventionally for- bidden women, often called *yoginis, dakinis,* or *dutis.* Such women were usually low-caste and were believed to embody Shakti, divine feminine "energy."

In the tenth to eleventh centuries, furthermore, *hatha yoga* or "yoga of forceful exertion," based largely on the *Shaiva Tantras,* emerged as yet another yoga system. Although many of the postural yoga systems dis- cussed in proceeding chapters claim to derive from or to be modern forms of hatha yoga, that claim cannot stand historical scrutiny. Hatha yoga did involve a variety of postures, but in preparation for "internal sexual practices"—that is, the tantric manipulation of the subtle body (Samuel 2008: 279, 336)—or for "curative" aims, for example destroying poi- sons (Singleton 2010: 29; Singleton cites the fifteenth–sixteenth-century *Hatha Yoga Pradipika* [I.33]). Furthermore, the methods and aims of hatha yoga, outlined below, would not be familiar to most contemporary practi- tioners of modern postural yoga.

Hatha yoga texts propound a notion of subtle physiology. The sub- tle body is composed of *nadis* or "veins" through which *prana* or subtle "breath" flows. A central technique is breath control, which serves to purify and balance the nadis and, in combination with other techniques, including postures and bodily *mudra* or "seals," awakens Shakti in the form of a serpent, *kundalini* (from Sanskrit, *kundala* or "to coil"), who otherwise lies dormant, coiled up at the bottom of the spine. The tech- niques of hatha yoga draw her up through the central nadi, and, as she moves upward, she penetrates each major *chakra* or "wheel," where subtle breath is concentrated, thus awakening the latent prana therein. Finally, she reaches the highest chakra at the top of the head, and this internal union results in samadhi.

This *kundalini yoga* often takes on erotic symbolism. The copulation of Shiva and Shakti represent the nondual nature of reality itself, and it is erotic energy, sometimes believed to be located in the concentrated sub- stance of sexual fluids, that is imagined as flowing from the bottom of the spine to the top of the spine, where the erotic union between Shakti and Shiva occurs. This is especially the case in some tantric traditions, where techniques of erotic visualization or ritual copulation are used for the sake of stimulating and then sublimating energy toward higher states of knowledge, culminating in the realization of nonduality.

Though hatha yoga does not "belong" to any single South Asian tradition (Mallinson 2005: 113), and there was significant exchange between the Shaiva Nath yoga tradition (circa twelfth century)—members of which made up the only South Asian order to self-identify as *yogis* (White 2012: 17)—and other yoga traditions, from Vaishnavas to Sufis, founders of the Nath tradition were hatha yoga's earliest systematizers.[19] The earliest and best-known texts of hatha yoga include the *Goraksha Sataka* (circa twelfth century), ascribed to Gorakshanatha; the *Shiva Samhita* (fifteenth century); the *Hatha Yoga Pradipika* (fifteenth–sixteenth century); the *Hatha Ratnavali* (seventeenth century); the *Gheranda Samhita* (seventeenth–eighteenth century); and the *Joga Pradipaka* (eighteenth century) (Singleton 2010: 28).

In addition to Hindu tantra, there were also Buddhist and Jain tantric systems. Looking closely at Buddhist tantra in India, Ronald Davidson (2002) suggests that socioeconomic developments in early medieval India strongly influenced the rise and shape of tantra. Davidson shows how socioeconomic and sociopolitical developments, including economic and patronage crises, a decline in women's economic participation, and the establishment of large monastic orders, influenced the Buddhist tradition that would come to serve as the foundational religiosities upon which Buddhist cultures in China, Tibet, and Japan would build (2002).

On Haribhadra's Jain *Yoga Drishti Samuccaya*, Christopher Key Chapple suggests that Haribhadra, a medieval Jain thinker, perceived competition with tantra and thus, mirroring some oppositional Vedantic responses to tantra, critiqued its transgressive dimensions while appropriating aspects of it that were seemingly compatible with Jain thought (Chapple 1998: 29; Chapple 2003: 85). Chapple suggests that a comparison between the earlier Jain *Yoga Bindu*, in which tantra is absent, and the later Jain *Yoga Drishti Samuccaya*, in which tantra is present, supports Samuel's argument that any account of yoga must acknowledge that it is a dynamic, perpetually changing phenomenon:

Presumably, Virahāṅka Haribhadra wrote the *Yogabindu* in the sixth century. This would account for its interest in Buddhism and its neglect of Tantra. Buddhism was still vital in India in the sixth century, and as we know from the legendary biographical accounts,

Haribhadra had perhaps been well-served by extending an olive branch to this competing tradition. Haribhadra Yākinī-Putra wrote the *Yogadṛṣṭisamuccaya* in the eighth century. This would account for the vituperative protests against the Tantric Kaula *yogīs* and the interest in engaging the Vedāntins in conversation. The author includes but places less emphasis on the Buddhists. Tantra was in its ascendancy and a direct competitor with Jainism in Gujarat, and Vedānta was in the process of revitalization and quickly gaining Buddhist converts. (Chapple 2011: 333)

As stated above, yoga never appeared independent of specific contexts. And, in tantric contexts especially, yoga systems that served soteriological purposes were also appropriated for the sake of meeting *bhukti* or mundane objectives, often of royal courts (Samuel 2008). According to Samuel:

> If we want to understand what early Śaiva Tantrics were doing, for example, it is surely relevant that they were probably doing it, much of the time, in the context of being employed as official sorcerers, healers and magical practitioners by local rulers and 'big men'...we have to see similar contexts for much Buddhist and Jaina Tantric practice as well...(Samuel 2011: 311)

The Shaiva Nath yoga tradition is especially known for the resources it offered such "big men," since hatha yoga functioned for them as a means to bodily immortality, sexual pleasure, as well as supernatural and sociopolitical powers (White 1996; White 2009). Such benefits were associated with yoga prior to the Nath tradition, but its members were the first to identify these benefits as the explicit aims of the yogi (White 2012: 17–18). Sometimes these aims were nefarious, and thus Nath Yogis had reputations as sinister villains (see White 2009).

Medieval Jain appropriations of tantra provide a demonstrative example of yoga's context-sensitivity when it came to the pursuit of mundane objectives. Overall, tantric thought and practice played minor roles in Jain traditions relative to Hindu and Buddhist ones. This is probably, in part, because Jains maintained a dualist metaphysics that was opposed to the nondualist metaphysics dominant in tantra (Dundas 2000; Qvarnström 2000). Nevertheless, even Jains, whose path toward salvation necessitated total renunciation of and disassociation from the material world, in the medieval period embraced tantric yoga by regarding it as a system of different means (sadhana) for attaining mundane objectives rather than as part of the path to salvation (Qvarnström 1998: 37).

Chapple evaluates Haribhadra and his "cosmopolitan" interest in tantric yoga (Chapple 1998: 15). Haribhadra placed yogic techniques in an "orthodox Jain framework" in an attempt to expand his audience (Chapple 1998: 20). Haribhadra both criticized the Kula yoga tradition for its antinomian practices but also appropriated certain of its tantric elements into his own form of Jain yoga in an attempt to "co-opt" its lure (Chapple 1998: 26).[20] Chapple explains:

> ...[Haribhadra] emphasizes the path of purity as the only true yogic means to liberation. However, he attempts this in a subtle fashion. Rather than setting forth the particular (and stringent) aspects of Jain purification practice, Haribhadra cloaks the Jain guṇasthāna system in the combined guise of Patanjali's Aṣṭānga Yoga and a Tantric Aṣṭa Mātṛkā system. Some of the names he employs are well-known as Hindu goddesses or yoginīs; others are close approximations. Through this device, and by introducing the text with a thinly veiled reference to the threefold emphasis on Desire, Study, and Practice in Tantric traditions, Haribhadra attempts to demonstrate that the heterodox movements offer nothing other than what already exists in the practice of his form of Jain Yoga. (Chapple 1998: 29; see also Chapple 2003: 85)

On the topic of medieval Jain appropriations of tantra, John E. Cort suggests Jains used *vidyas*, multiword magical spells or invocations presided over by female deities and learnt by initiation and practicing the prescribed sadhana (Cort 1987: 237). Such vidyas were used for the sake of mundane objectives, not for progress along the path toward salvation (Cort 1987: 238). Likewise, Paul Dundas and Cort demonstrate how Shaiva transferences to Jain thought occurred during the medieval period, particularly in the development of a Jain *mantra shastra* and the attendant rituals for the sake of gaining magical powers (Dundas 1998; Cort 2000: 417; Dundas 2000: 232).

Whereas Hindu and Buddhist schools incorporated tantric practices into their soteriologies, Jain schools incorporated tantra only as a secondary tradition aimed at worldly goals rather than the goal of salvation, and thus tantra did not threaten orthodox soteriological doctrine (Cort

1987: 238–239; Qvarnström 1998: 37; Cort 2000: 417). In other words, we do not find a tantric path to salvation in Jain tantra. Rather, the Jain ascetic path remains the path to salvation, although Jain appropriations of tantra demonstrate that Jains maintained a concern not just with salvation from the world, but also with worldly goals (Cort 2000: 417). Such appropriations were for the sake of "co-opting" tantra's popularity in order to adapt to the social climate of medieval South Asia, where the presence of tantra made certain religious complexes more attractive to large audiences (Chapple 1998; Qvarnström 1998: 40).

Conclusion

By the end of the first millennium c.e., yoga systems were widespread in South Asia, and Hindu, Buddhist, and Jain textual traditions prescribed them. Following the twelfth-century Muslim incursions into South Asia and the establishment of Islam as a South Asian religion, Sufis appropriated elements of yoga into their mystical thought and practice (see, e.g., Ernst 2012). Therefore, throughout its history in South Asia, yoga was culturally South Asian but did not belong to any single religious tradition. In the history of yoga leading up to the nineteenth century, rather than essentializing yoga by reifying its content and aims, it is more accurate to identify it as heterogeneous in practice and characteristic of the doctrinally diverse premodern culture of South Asia.

Reflecting on recent research (specifically Davidson 2002 and Samuel 2008) that emphasizes the significant role of social contexts in shaping yoga systems, Vesna Wallace reiterates the need for a contextual understanding of yoga: "the socio-political environments of the Yogic and Tantric practices at some point became replicated in the structures of these practices and determined their social values," and "certain social principles that guide religious practices can become transformed and in some cases even nullified in response to historical and sociopolitical contexts" (Wallace 2011: 336). In short, yoga is contextual. I suggest we consider this the most notable lesson from the study of premodern yoga to consider as we approach the study of modern yoga.

Images of yoga from the premodern world, whether of philosopher-ascetics turning inward in pursuit of salvation through realization of the true self, ecstatic *bhaktas* or devotees turning outward in pursuit of divine union with Krishna, or sinister villains channeling bodily energy in pursuit of sexual pleasure, are hardly the images that we tend to envision when we think of modern practitioners of yoga. In other words, modern yoga systems, including postural yoga ones, bear little resemblance to the yoga systems that preceded them. This is because what modern yoga systems do share with premodern ones is that they are specific to their own social contexts. It is to the contexts of early modern yoga that I now turn.

2

From Counterculture to Counterculture

> *To the average uninstructed man or woman, there is no apparent relation between the honeymoon and that philosophy which I prefer to call "yoga." And yet, if yoga were properly understood and practiced in the marital embrace by every newly married couple, their sex life would be, from the start, so holy, so healthy, so happy, that they would never care to descend to the methods commonly practiced among married people today.*
>
> —IDA C. CRADDOCK, *The Wedding Night* (1900: 213)

THE HISTORY OF modern yoga is a history of divergence, debate, exclusion, and controversy, as well as assimilation, inclusion, and collectivity. As noted in Chapter One, the systematic construction and practice of premodern yoga in South Asia, dating back to around two thousand years ago, were also complex. Yoga was a tradition made up of heterogeneous systems of thought and practice in which individuals sought to destabilize normal consciousness and ways of experiencing or manipulating the world. Sometimes, yoga techniques were believed to cultivate mystical states of consciousness characterized by knowledge of ultimate reality, and for the most advanced adepts, to eventually result in salvation from suffering existence. Other times, yoga techniques were believed to cultivate supernatural powers or to facilitate the pursuit of mundane objectives. For much of its premodern history, yoga was culturally pervasive throughout South Asia and did not belong to any single religious tradition, such as the Hindu, Buddhist, or

Jain traditions. So in premodern South Asia, rather than identify it with one particular tradition, it is more accurate to identify it as characteristic of the doctrinally and practically diverse South Asian religious culture.

Beginning in the nineteenth century, however, yoga was deconstructed and reconstructed both within and beyond South Asia, leading to the emergence of a new transnational tradition. That tradition is modern yoga, which is made up of heterogeneous systems that developed as a consequence of encounters between Indian yoga reformers engaged with modern thought, Europeans and Americans interested in topics ranging from metaphysics to fitness, and modern sociopolitical phenomena. Although, in the popular imagination, yoga's global diffusion beyond India is associated with the counterculture of the 1960s and especially the Beatles, well before the 1960s yogis across the globe participated in countercultural movements in which they practiced and disseminated their innovative renditions of modern yoga.

The subject of this chapter is the early history of modern yoga from the nineteenth century to the middle of the twentieth century. Understanding the early history of modern yoga is key to understanding how the late twentieth century serves as a new phase of development in the history of yoga and, more specifically, postural yoga. Unsurprisingly, as globalization and transnational cultural products emerged in the nineteenth century, primarily as a consequence of the dominant socioeconomic forces of market capitalism, colonial and industrial endeavors, and the concomitant rapid cultural changes among both colonizing and colonized populations, yoga became subject to processes of translation and accommodation as its proponents actively modernized it. I will demonstrate that, with all of the divergences that make up this early history of modern yoga, the data reinforce a collective historical pattern: Modern yoga, until the second half of the twentieth century, was made up of controversial, elite, or countercultural movements opposed to prevailing religious orthodoxies. Thus modern yoga went global but did not yet represent a pop culture product, something embraced by the general populace. By demonstrating that the history of modern yoga is not so simplistic as a linear trajectory of increasing global popularization, this chapter will establish an important premise to my argument in proceeding chapters that certain social changes in the middle of the twentieth century enabled the shift of modern yoga from counterculture to pop culture.

Controversy and Censorship

I begin with the most tragic controversy in the history of modern yoga as it developed around the figure of Ida C. Craddock (1857–1902).[1] I begin with Craddock because the life of this American yogi serves as a model for identifying recurrent themes in the early history of modern yoga, especially the extent to which modern yoga was either feared and loathed by or perceived as foreign to mainstream populations across the globe.

To understand why Craddock was feared and loathed, one must understand her social and historical context. This was a period of religious questioning in the United States in light of emergent modern historical and scientific analyses that challenged the dominant Christian orthodox ideas about the way the world was and why it was that way. Perhaps the most palpable example of modern challenges to religious orthodoxy was Darwin's theory of evolution, which put into question orthodox Christian doctrine on creation and history. Whereas some responded to such modern challenges to orthodoxy by constructing new religions that assimilated aspects of various worldviews, including Asian and modern scientific ones, others responded with religious fundamentalism.[2] Of particular significance to the history of modern yoga is Evangelical Protestant Christianity, which functioned as the cultural and legal standard in the United States at the turn of the century.[3] Many socially and politically influential individuals and organizations used that standard to actively suppress what were deemed intolerable religious ideas and practices, including those of early modern yogis.

In the United States, there were various attempts to legally enforce fundamentalist interpretations of what it meant to be a "Christian nation." Most notable were those of United States Postal Inspector Anthony Comstock (1844–1915). Comstock founded the New York Society for the Suppression of Vice and used his position in the postal service to censor whatever he deemed a threat to the fundamentalist Protestant Christian morals he identified as American. Comstock worked with law enforcement, the media, and the Christian clergy to harass and often bring legal cases against those he deemed a moral threat to American society, including Craddock.[4] His attacks on all things deemed threatening included a condemnation of yoga, especially its body practices. His normative religious standard was characterized by a subordination of the body to the soul, and it especially denounced sexual pleasure, which it considered an obstacle to spiritual development.

Craddock was the antithesis to that standard. Having refuted the prevailing mainstream argument that women should not participate in scholarship, she established herself as an independent scholar of "Phallic Worship" in the history of religions. It was in the context of her scholarship that she encountered the esoteric tantric components of hatha yoga.[5] Craddock accessed *The Esoteric Science and Philosophy of the Tantras, Shiva Sanhita*, an English translation of one of the earliest and best-known texts of hatha yoga, the *Shiva Samhita* (fifteenth century). In that text, Craddock found the idea that sexual union could facilitate divine realization and key techniques, most notably the *vajroli mudra*. In Hindu tantra, the *vajroli mudra* or "urethral suction" required the male partner in sexual intercourse to exercise control over ejaculation and functioned as a hydraulic technique through which male and female sexual fluids were transformed within the male body in order to bring about "an immortal yet concrete *diamond body* that transcends the laws of nature" (White 1996: 72). Craddock reconstructed those components of tantra into a system of techniques, most importantly delayed ejaculation, for enhancing sexual pleasures within the boundaries of marriage and simultaneously advancing the state of the soul in relation to God. Though the secrets revealed in the *Shiva Samhita* were initially intended for a small audience, Craddock had no interest in such secrecy. According to Leigh Schmidt:

> The mysterious veiling commanded in *The Esoteric Science and Philosophy of the Tantras* was lost on Craddock. If these teachings were "hidden and kept secret in all the TANTRAS," that was not a confidence she was at all interested in preserving. Such tight-lipped rules were utterly contrary to the frankness of speech and freedom of expression for which American marriage reformers were fighting. (Schmidt 2010: 129–130)

Inspired by the mystico-erotic techniques of tantra, she prescribed seminal retention during heterosexual intercourse in order to enhance the pleasures experienced by women and men.[6] And in a creative redefinition of tantra's sacralization of sexual union, Craddock constructed a new vision of sexual intercourse between married women and men that considered God to be a third partner in what amounted to a sacred *ménage à trois*.

In addition to yoga's significance to Craddock's mystico-erotic religion, it was also at the center of her public persona from the time she established the Church of Yoga in 1899. She increasingly incited rage among those who opposed her socioreligious and sexual reform agenda. Consequently, there were tensions between Craddock and government officials who sought to enforce legal standards that would qualify her radical agenda as illegally obscene and blasphemous. In 1902, after being convicted in a New York trial for such charges, Craddock spent three torturous months in prison. After her release, an upcoming federal trial threatened additional prison time. Craddock responded by taking her own life in order to die a free woman.

So in what ways does the life of this radical American yogi-sexologist reveal important themes in the early history of modern yoga? The first has to do with the role of the human body in modern yoga. Even though Craddock's sacralization of sexual intercourse is not radical by today's popular American standards and, in Leigh Schmidt's words, may even seem "mundane" to the contemporary reader, for the mainstream turn-of-the-century American, it was antisocial heterodoxy (Schmidt 2010: 273). This demonstrates that not only was the sacralization of the body present in this early system of modern yoga, but it was also so significant to that system that martyrdom occurred on its behalf. In many articulations of modern yoga, some of which will be discussed below, body practices were censored for the same reasons Craddock had to sacrifice her life for them.

Which brings us to the second theme. Craddock's story reveals the extent to which turn-of-the-century mainstream populations feared modern yoga, especially when it emphasized various body practices. Modern yoga was not generally welcomed by mainstream populations, but instead was often deemed a threat to prevailing religious and social orthodoxies. And although there was never a stark bifurcation between the physical techniques and the meditative techniques of yoga prior to the modern period, since the turn of the century such a bifurcation has permeated transnational discourse on yoga. Although, as we will see below, many countercultural movements that embraced the psychological and intellectual components of yoga or what was often termed *raja yoga* were also disliked by much of the mainstream populations from India to the United States, those who were interested in and engaged in physical techniques faced the harshest criticisms.[7]

Third, Craddock's construction of yoga is consistent with the history of modern yoga's saturation with processes of adaptation, assimilation, and syncretism. Craddock identified as a Unitarian but also as the pastor of the Church of Yoga. The fact that a woman could be so polymorphously religious reflects the realities of modernity and its pluralizing processes, but it also reflects yoga's malleability. In other words, yoga at the turn of the century was something that certain countercultural individuals deemed capable of adaptation, assimilation, and syncretism.

Pierre Bernard (1876–1955) was another famously adaptive, assimilative, and syncretic figure in the early history of modern yoga.[8] Like Craddock, he was a turn-of-the-century American social radical and tantric yogi. But unlike Craddock, his fate was not so grim. Whereas those who feared Craddock thwarted her dissemination of yoga, Bernard succeeded in training a number of American disciples who continued to practice and teach yoga throughout the country well into the second half of the twentieth century.[9]

Bernard discovered yoga in his boyhood when he met an Indian yogi by the name of Sylvais Hamati (dates unknown) in Lincoln, Nebraska. Hamati became Bernard's guru and taught him hatha yoga techniques. Bernard spent years reveling in the public spectacle of his yogic trances that apparently were so deep that doctors could thread needles through his face without even causing him to flinch. In later years, he became a fashionable businessman and community leader. He was at once charismatic, generous, mysterious, and deceitful.

At every stage of Bernard's yoga career, mainstream Americans remained suspicious of his teachings. Furthermore, he did not witness the popularization of modern yoga in his lifetime. For these reasons, Bernard only attracted a small following made up of those who could afford, both financially and socially, to be eccentric. And despite the numerous attempts by law enforcement, the media, and the Christian clergy to force Bernard and his students to forfeit yoga, they resisted.

But it was not easy. Bernard struggled to construct a public persona as a man of science and scholarship, although he held no degrees from any higher-education institution. For years, he and his students were run out of city after city (as far as London, where one of his closest disciples attempted to recruit students and was consequently deported by British authorities). In New York City in 1910, there were accusations that Bernard was involved in the "white slave trade" and, more specifically, was forcing young women to engage in antinomian sexual practices. While awaiting trial for the alleged crimes, he was imprisoned in "the Tombs," a New York City prison famous for its horrific living conditions, for three-and-a-half months. The only evidence in support of the accusations was the testimony of two of his former disciples, so he was released when those disciples suddenly dropped all charges and fled the state.

Finally, in 1918, Bernard and his disciples settled in Nyack, New York, where Bernard built an esoteric country club for "tantriks" (practitioners of tantra) that flourished for years thanks to the abundant financial support of rich and famous individuals and families, most noteworthy of which were members of the Vanderbilt family. Clients came to Bernard's club to learn his rendition of hatha yoga, which he promised would enhance their pleasures in life, as well as to enjoy the opulent circuses and other celebrations hosted by Bernard and his disciples.

All of this reflects Bernard's life-affirming rendition of yoga. He constructed yoga anew by combining the physical techniques of modern hatha yoga—as detailed below, this form of hatha yoga was influenced by modern physical culture—the erotico-mysticism of tantra, and a communal ethic based on his nondualist philosophy. Yoga, according to Bernard, enabled people to enhance their physical health and pleasures and thus experience a life lived well. Bernard supplemented yoga by enhancing the pleasures of life at the club in every way he could. Unlike many of his modern yoga contemporaries in the United States, including numerous Indian gurus, such as Swami Vivekananda (more on Vivekananda below), who disseminated ascetic, intellectual, and meditational renditions of yoga, Bernard was a guru of immanent means to an immanent aim: pleasure. For that very reason, given the puritanical mores that dominated his social world, he had to keep much of his yoga system secret.

And there were other European and American yogis who kept their interests in and practice of yoga secret for fear that they would stir controversy and perhaps even direct conflict. Sir John Woodroffe (1865–1936), a British High Court Judge in Calcutta, was another esoteric modern yogi of this variety.[10] Woodroffe studied tantric texts, selected from the *Tantras*, probably translated by his Bengali friend and pundit Atul Behari Ghose (1864–1936). For Woodroffe, tantra was a scholarly interest as well as a personal one. In fact, it is possible he underwent tantric initiation under the guidance of a guru and may have also participated in other esoteric tantric rituals. Under the pen-name *Arthur Avalon*, which, in addition to keeping his identity secret, may have functioned to represent the figures of both Woodroffe and Ghose, a number of texts on hatha yoga and tantra were published, including *The Serpent Power: The Secrets of Tantric and Shaktic Yoga* (1919). That text became a major English-language resource on such topics for countercultural religious groups in North America and Europe throughout the twentieth century.

It turns out that, in addition to American and European countercultural yogis such as Craddock, Bernard, and Woodroffe, many nineteenth- and early-twentieth-century Indian yogis were also subject to serious and persistent criticisms for their interests in and practice of yoga. Their stories show a very different part of modern yoga's history from the one Vivekananda's visit to the United States conveys. More than anything else, a bifurcation between yogic meditative, philosophical, and ethical dimensions, prescribed by Vivekananda and associated with what has often been termed *classical yoga* or *raja* ("royal") *yoga*, and the physical techniques associated with hatha yoga affected the perception of yoga practitioners. The extreme hostility toward Craddock, Bernard, Woodroffe, and Indian proponents of hatha yoga as compared to the more subdued hostility toward proponents of raja yoga reflects the fact that, despite what one might suspect given the prevalence of postural yoga in pop culture today, modern yoga's early history shows that involvement in physical yoga cost a person more social currency than involvement in yoga focused on meditation, philosophy, or ethics.

An especially deep suspicion of those Indian yogis engaged in body practices was dominant among European, American, and Indian social and intellectual elites. Following the onset of British colonialism in India, elites from the United States, Europe, and India dismissed Indian systems of hatha yoga as extreme, barbaric, and antisocial practices. British colonialists and Christian missionaries, along with those Indian elites who sympathized with either or both causes, thought of hatha yoga as a backward and savage religion.

Much of that denunciation was fueled in the nineteenth century by widespread stereotypes about hatha yoga. First, abilities to contort the body into what were considered bizarre yoga postures, techniques associated with hatha yoga, were also associated with those abilities of Western contortionists (Singleton 2010: 57–59). Consequently, the physical techniques of hatha yoga were reduced to mere crass entertainment. Second, the supposed *siddhis* or magical powers of some such yogis resulted in the association of hatha yoga with occult magic (Singleton 2010: 64–66). Most scandalous of all, as a result of Aleister Crowley's (1875–1947) experiments with tantra, it became associated with sex magic (Urban 2006: 111). Hugh B. Urban suggests,

> Indian mysticism was imagined as something otherworldly and identified with Vedānta or other philosophical schools... Tantra represented, for both Indian and European authors, mysticism in its most degenerate form: a kind of mysticism that had been corrupted with sensual desire and this-worldly power. (Urban 2003: 15n53)

Because the "degenerate" vision of tantra included yoga's body practices, as opposed to the philosophical dimensions of Vedanta and other more widely respected schools of Indian thought, those techniques were most disdained in the early history of modern yoga. And because they received widespread attention in the writings of travelers, journalists, and scholars, derogatory visions came to represent hatha yoga to mainstream Europeans, Americans, and Indians. Mass-circulation writings on yoga reified colonialist and Orientalist conceptions of hatha yoga as particularly mysterious, bizarre, uncivilized, and threatening to modernity and rationality. Mark Singleton describes the situation: "As mass-circulation print media brought images of yogic austerities to a wider audience, the *hatha* yogin's reputation as the eccentric extreme of the Indian religious spectrum was increasingly cemented" (Singleton 2010: 56).

Modern Yoga from the Neck Up

Participants in various modernizing movements, however, were interested in salvaging yoga from its reputation as a system of extreme, antisocial practices and instead establishing its legitimacy as a philosophical, meditational, or ethical tradition. They reflected a general trend in the nineteenth- and early-twentieth-century global religious landscape. As mentioned above, this was a period of religious questioning in light of modernity. In response to new questions about the nature of the body, the soul, and the mind, metaphysical, philosophical, and social movements arose, motivated by the desire to redefine the relationship between these three constituents of the human being. Transcendentalism, Theosophy, New Thought, Christian Science, and the Vedanta Society as well as Indian reform movements, including the Brahmo Samaj and the Ramakrishna Mission, were some of the most notable movements that assimilated and syncretized ideas and practices from Christian Protestantism, modern science, yoga and other South Asian traditions, and sometimes Mind

Cure, a new healing system that invoked the power of the mind over the body in order to treat illness.

In the various attempts by members of such movements to construct systems of yoga deemed compatible with their modern agendas, they elided certain aspects of yoga and emphasized others. Because of hatha yoga and tantra's associations with what were considered bizarre yoga postures, extreme asceticism, magic, sexual obscenity, and popular entertainment, they did not take them seriously. Instead, in various ways, they all emphasized the ethical, philosophical, or meditational components of yoga associated with so-called classical yoga or raja yoga. Many of the movements that only assimilated those aspects of yoga were less subject to controversy than figures like Craddock and Bernard because they censored yoga of its most scandalous practices. European and American individuals and organizations who remained on the side of Christian orthodoxy, and especially those energized by a new fundamentalist ideology, however, still thought such movements were a danger to all they considered decent, pure, and godly.

American Transcendentalists, for example, most significantly Ralph Waldo Emerson (1803–1882) and Henry David Thoreau (1817–1862), were deemed threatening to Christian orthodoxy when they valorized yoga's ethical and meditational dimensions.[11] They encountered yoga by reading Indian literature, particularly the *Bhagavad Gita*, and their interests were primarily in what they perceived to be the intellectual components of yoga. The Transcendentalists thought their democratic religiosity that privileged unmediated intuition as a means to the realization of God was compatible with nondualist Indian thought that maintained that knowledge of ultimate reality could be discovered through a yogic process of turning inward, away from the external world of doctrine. Transcendentalist thought countered and, therefore, was perceived as a threat to mainstream American religious values, which deemed God to be outward, beyond the world and the self, rather than inward, immanently present within the self. For this reason, Emerson was ostracized from his alma mater, Harvard University, after his famous "Divinity School Address" (1838) in which he shared his Transcendentalist vision.

Some quasi-unorthodox European intellectuals also valorized the intellectual components of yoga while simultaneously criticizing the physical practices of hatha yoga. The Oxford University Indologist, Max Muller (1823–1900), for example, criticized:

[the] tortures which some of them, who hardly deserve to be called Samnyasins, for they are not much better than jugglers or Hathayogins, inflict on themselves, the ascetic methods by which they try to subdue and annihilate their passions, and bring themselves to a state of extreme nervous exaltation accompanied by trances or fainting fits of long duration. (Muller 1974 [1898]: vii)

At the same time, Muller valorized yoga in its "early stages," when it "was truly philosophical" before he believed it degenerated into practical systems, worst of which was hatha yoga (Muller 1899: 407, 465, quoted in Singleton 2010: 43).[12] Another esteemed Oxford University Indologist, Monier Monier-Williams (1819–1899), shared Muller's contempt for hatha yoga, describing it as "a strange compound of mental and bodily exercises, consisting [of] unnatural restraint, forced and painful postures, twisting and contortions of the limbs, suppression of the breath and utter absence of mind" (quoted in Love 2010: 73).

The Theosophical Society, founded in New York City in 1875, shared such intellectuals' contempt for hatha yoga.[13] Helena Blavatsky (1831–1891), co-founder of the Theosophical Society, and other members consistently criticized hatha yoga, although they were not opposed to all yoga systems. In fact, it was the Theosophical Society that first reified the notion of raja yoga, which would come to be identified with classical yoga, by equating it with a narrow philosophical and meditational tradition based on a selective reading of the *Yoga Sutras* (de Michelis 2004: 178). They even arranged for the publication of an English translation of the *Yoga Sutras*, the source most widely cited on classical yoga to this day. On the one hand, they considered the physical techniques associated with hatha yoga to be inferior forms of practice (de Michelis 2004: 178). Even breathing, according to Blavatsky, was a backward yogic practice and:

...pertains to the lower Yoga. The *Hatha* so called was and still is discountenanced by the Arhats. It is injurious to the health and alone can never develop into Raja Yoga. (Blavatsky 1888: 95; see also de Michelis 2004: 178; Albanese 2007: 351; Singleton 2010: 76–77)

In Blavatsky's thought, raja yoga, in contrast to hatha yoga, was a valuable meditational and philosophical yoga system. She equated it not only with Patanjala Yoga, but also with the *jnana yoga* or the "yoga of knowledge" of Shankara's *advaita vedanta* or "nondual vedanta" school as well as with modern "hypnotism" and "self-mesmerisation" (de Michelis 2004: 178).[14]

Another Theosophist, William Judge (1851–1896), provided a commentary on the *Yoga Sutras* in which he continued along the same lines as Blavatsky, emphatically distinguishing between hatha yoga and raja yoga and warning of the dangers of hatha yoga's physical techniques, which he believed were "not spiritual" (Albanese 2007: 352). In light of Judge's condemnations, Catherine Albanese suggests, "What appealed to a late-nineteenth-century Anglo-American about the *Yoga Sutras*, we can guess, was the moral inscription that the text—and Judge's presentation of it—wrote over yogic practice" (Albanese 2007: 352). In other words, Americans and Europeans elided those aspects of yoga that were not compatible with their own modern intellectual, ethical, and religious ideas and practices and emphasized those on which they could project their own modern agendas.

But Europeans and Americans were not the only ones who reified and privileged a notion of raja yoga that censored the physical practices associated with hatha yoga and that was perceived to be compatible with modern ideas and values, especially a modern interpretation of advaita vedanta or neo-vedanta, which interpreted nondualism as a rational Indian philosophical religion based on self-development and ethical activism. Reid Locklin and Julia Lauwers note two opposing Indian responses to the global diffusion of advaita vedanta (2009). On the one hand, various forms of Indian religious nationalisms that emphasized geocentric national identity, such as that of the Rashtriya Swayamsevak Sangh (RSS) and the Vishwa Hindu Parishad (VHP), resisted global diffusion (Locklin and Lauwers 2009). On the other hand, accommodationist approaches, such as that of Vivekananda and Swami Chinmayananda (1916–1993), actively pursued global diffusion by emphasizing Hindu universalism and deemphasizing caste and national identity (Locklin and Lauwers 2009). Accommodationist approaches to yoga sought to revive advaita vedanta for Indians and to simultaneously promote it as a universally accessible gift to humanity (Locklin and Lauwers 2009). Accommodationists accomplished this mission by presenting advaita vedanta in the modern "universalist, objective language of natural science, meditative technique, and spiritual therapy" (Locklin and Lauwers 2009: 183).

More than any European or American, the famous Hindu proselytizing guru Vivekananda was responsible for systematizing and globally diffusing a narrow and modern version of yoga. Vivekananda was one among many Hindus who expressed contempt for certain types of yoga based on a bifurcation between yoga's philosophical and meditative techniques, often equated with raja yoga, and its physical techniques, often equated with hatha yoga (Singleton 2010: 44–49, 70–80).

De Michelis, who suggests that Vivekananda was the "creator" of "Modern Yoga," argues that he was responsible for starting "something of a 'yoga renaissance' both in India and in the West" (de Michelis 2004: 1–9, 90, 182). He did this through the diffusion of a modern notion of raja yoga. Vivekananda used *raja yoga* to refer to what he considered authentic yoga according to his selective reading of the *Yoga Sutras*. Vivekananda was the founder of the Ramakrishna Mission, an Indian organization that promoted a modern interpretation of advaita vedanta, and advocated for the spirituality of Indian culture as opposed to the so-called materialism of Western culture. Vivekananda and his Ramakrishna Mission served as models of the Orientalist stereotype of India. In Richard King's words,

> In Vivekānanda's hands, Orientalist notions of India as 'other worldly' and 'mystical' were embraced and praised as India's special gift to humankind. Thus the very discourse that succeeded in alienating, subordinating and controlling India was used by Vivekānanda as a religious clarion call for the Indian people to unite under the banner of a universalistic and all-embracing Hinduism. (King 1999: 93)

Under the influence of colonialist, Orientalist, Christian missionary, and Theosophical condemnations of hatha yoga, Vivekananda sought to disseminate a form of yoga to "the West" that would be perceived as the antithesis to the body-centered religion popularly associated with yoga. His first visit to the United States came in 1893 with his famous speech to the Parliament of the World's Religions in Chicago, in which he described the Hindu tradition in a way that portrayed it as an experiential, not doctrinaire, philosophy that was compatible with the ideals of modernity.[15] This charismatic guru impressed many in the audience, and his appearance at the Parliament initiated a series of lecture tours throughout the United States.

A number of Vivekananda's qualities appealed to certain segments of the American and South Asian populations. Vivekananda especially appealed to American women interested in alternatives to orthodox religion. The guru joined Transcendentalists, Theosophists, and Hindu reformers in projecting modern values and ideas onto a reified notion of Hinduism. The result, for Vivekananda, was a modern and nondualist interpretation of Patanjala Yoga, and with his book entitled *Raja Yoga* (1896) and other texts, Vivekananda and the Ramakrishna Mission ossified the equation of raja yoga with a modern and nondualist interpretation of Patanjala Yoga by providing it with indigenous authority.[16]

For something to qualify as modern, it had to be compatible with science, so Vivekananda sought to prove that raja yoga was scientific. In this context, he did invoke some components of hatha yoga, but only on his own terms. Basically, he appropriated the notion of the subtle body, which he argued had correspondences in the physical body as mapped out in modern anatomy and physiology (de Michelis 2004: 166–167). In this way, he argued, subtle energy could function as a healing agent (de Michelis 2004: 163–168). Health benefits, however, were inferior to what he considered the true aim of yoga: spiritual development (Vivekananda 1992 [1896]: 20).

Furthermore, while acknowledging that yogic metaphysics and meditation could have implications for the physical body, he largely rejected the physical practices associated with hatha yoga. In fact, on the topic of hatha yoga practices, he insisted, "we have nothing to do with it here, because its practices are very difficult, and cannot be learned in a day, and, after all, do not lead to much spiritual growth" (Vivekananda 1992 [1896]: 20). Vivekananda focused instead on what he perceived to be the psychological benefits of yoga and an emphasis on the self that would be perceived as compatible with the modern democratic emphasis on the individual, and ignored those aspects of yoga that were perceived as nonrational.

Vivekananda's elision of yoga's body practices was not an isolated incident of censorship in Vivekananda's life but reflected a larger pattern. As demonstrated by Jeffrey J. Kripal and Hugh B. Urban, Vivekananda also censored the hagiography of his guru, Ramakrishna (1836–1886), by selectively eliding those references that revealed the guru's engagement with hatha yoga and especially tantra (Kripal 1998; Urban 2003). Such things were apparently too countercultural for Vivekananda's taste. He probably also perceived them as incompatible with his desire for the global diffusion and universal application of Hindu thought.[17]

And yet, simultaneously, in a countercultural move akin to that of Emerson and other Transcendentalists, Vivekananda encouraged his disciples to turn inward, toward the self, rather than outward, toward either Christian or Hindu orthodox doctrine. He took the modern version of advaita vedanta and prescribed it as a universal religion that he believed was rational, practical, scientific, progressive, utilitarian, and psychological (de Michelis 2004: 91, 119). Echoing Muller's conception of the history of yoga, Vivekananda claimed that any version of yoga other than the one he prescribed was a corruption of its true, original form, arguing, "From the time it was discovered, more than four thousand years ago, Yoga was perfectly delineated, formulated and preached in India" (Vivekananda 1992 [1896]: 20).

Vivekananda's approach to yoga was a nondualist one aimed toward enhancing life in the world, but not in the same ways that figures like Craddock or Bernard had in mind. Vivekananda, himself a celibate monk, was not concerned with enhancing the pleasures of the body, but with enhancing life through a psychological process requiring self-control and meditation.

Vivekananda's emphasis on meditation and self-realization appealed to many countercultural Americans who rejected mainstream institutional forms of Protestant Christianity for new metaphysical movements, such as Christian Science and New Thought. Vivekananda and these Americans were all interested in wedding metaphysics with modern ideas and values as well as the aim of self-realization.[18] Attracted to his individualistic and democratic religious teachings, these Americans welcomed Vivekananda as a teacher, and he in turn responded to their desires and needs. As articulated by Elizabeth de Michelis, "This pattern of social interaction continued throughout his stay in the West: embraced by the more fluid, unchurched, affluent strands of the cultic milieu, he in turn adapted to them" (de Michelis 2004: 114). In all of these ways, Vivekananda appealed to an American audience made up of individuals with largely unorthodox religious interests, though they were unwilling to go so far as to embrace the most controversial of yoga practices popularly associated with hatha yoga.

Vivekananda prescribed yoga in a form that differed dramatically from those of more controversial early modern yogis, such as Craddock and Bernard. Craddock and Bernard's renditions of yoga even resulted in persecution because they were interested in the physical practices that could result in more pleasurable experiences of the body. Vivekananda censored yoga of the physical practices that were most sacred to Craddock and Bernard and most despised by American, Western European, and Indian intellectual and social elites. Because he prescribed an ascetic, Protestant yoga, he was successful in establishing a network of American centers for what he called the Vedanta Society, an organization for the dissemination of yoga. In his attempt to contrast Craddock with Vivekananda, Schmidt illuminates the approach to the body in Vivekananda's yoga:

> While the swami's emphasis on focused meditation connected nicely with Craddock's New Thought leanings, his body talk was hardly conducive to her sex-reform gospel. A proponent of chastity and renunciation, Vivekananda characterized his relationship to women in desexualized, child-like terms and consistently glossed over the eroticized mysticism of his own sainted guru, Ramakrishna, in favor of a more abstractly universalistic philosophy. In many ways Vivekananda actually stood as something of a Comstockian censor of Hindu traditions, hiding the bodily concerns and anxieties of his own teacher behind a veil of pure spirituality. That meditative version of yoga—no body-twisting postures, no openly erotic content—certainly helped Vivekananda make his Vedanta Society a relatively palatable offering in the American religious marketplace. (Schmidt 2010: 125)

Yet despite its opposition to the controversial body-centered yoga techniques, the Vedanta Society and its members were still marginalized by the American mainstream, which perceived yoga in all its forms to be a threat to social mores. Robert Love describes the Society:

> It was all very polite. The yoga the Vedantists taught was mental exercise—yoga from the neck up—and it went over very well in the hushed parlors of Back Bay, Fifth Avenue, and Lake Shore Drive. Any controversy it provoked derived not from scandals of the flesh, but from the domestic frenzy that ensued when its most fervent American converts followed the trail of incense to its logical end and renounced all worldly desires, in some cases breaking ties with husbands, wives, children, and family fortunes. (Love 2010: 72)

Yoga, in all its varieties, eventually developed such a bad reputation in the United States, especially for what were considered its ascetic challenges to marriage—there was clearly a misogynist thread to the criticism—that in 1909, even the Theosophical Society banned all conversation on yoga. Annie Besant (1847–1933), president of the American Theosophical Society at that time, went so far as to describe women who were practicing yoga as "animalistic" (Author unknown 1909b: 8; see also Author unknown 1909a: 3). A 1911 headline in a *Washington Post* Sunday special on the variety of controversies surrounding American yogis succinctly evidences the general identification of yoga with the antithesis of American social mores:

> This Soul Destroying Poison of the East: The Tragic Flood of Broken Homes and Hearts, Disgrace and Suicide That Follows the Broadening Stream of Morbidly Alluring Oriental 'Philosophies' into Our Country (Author unknown 1911c: M6)

Soon, the United States government began an investigation of various yogis to reveal just how many Americans, especially American women, had been seduced and cheated by yoga (Author unknown 1911a: 538; Author unknown 1911b: 20). By censoring yoga of the body, Vivekananda and his Society had developed a substantive following, but it was still perceived as a countercultural one in some parts of the world, to say the least.

Modern Yoga from the Neck Down

Today most people associate yoga with postural yoga, a fitness regimen that engages the physical body, mostly from the neck down. Yet this chapter on the early history of modern yoga is yet to reveal how postural yoga developed. Even figures like Craddock and Bernard, though they embraced yoga's physical techniques as one part of yoga practice, did not equate those techniques with fitness alone. They were also interested in the metaphysical manipulation of subtle energies and combined postures with nonphysical yoga techniques, all of which were associated with hatha yoga and, more specifically, tantra. Furthermore, the majority of early modern yogis, most significantly Vivekananda, despised body practices altogether.

The heterogeneity of systems that make up the history of modern yoga and the contrast between a disdain for body practices and a valorization of them in that history is exemplified by comparing Vivekananda to S. K. Pattabhi Jois (1915–2009). As described above, at the turn of the century, Vivekananda argued that the body practices associated with yoga had nothing to do with the true aim of yoga. In the middle of the twentieth century, however, Jois was one among many yoga proponents who became globally famous for prescribing yoga as a physical fitness regimen, primarily organized around posture practice. His emphasis on posture practice departed not just from the early history of modern yoga, but also from the history of yoga in general. In other words, posture practice was not central to any yoga tradition prior to the twentieth century.[19] So if postural yoga was not a direct continuation of something in the early history of modern yoga, and neither was it a revival of some premodern yoga system, the question arises: What occurred in the gap between Vivekananda and Jois that explains postural yoga's emergence and development?

Contemporary scholars, most notably Singleton (2010), have set about answering that question. In response to early-twentieth-century transnational ideas and movements, including military calisthenics (Sjoman 1996), modern medicine (Alter 2004), and the Western European and American physical culture of gymnasts, bodybuilders, martial experts, and contortionists (de Michelis 2004; Singleton 2010), modern yoga proponents ignited a passion for hatha yoga by constructing new postural yoga systems.[20] Postural yoga emerged "as a hybridized product of colonial India's dialogical encounter with the worldwide physical culture movement" (Singleton 2010: 80).

The methods of postural yoga were specific to the time period and would not have been considered yoga prior to this period of Indian history (Singleton 2010: 177). In fact, postural yoga was the "cultural successor [of] established methods of stretching and relaxing" that were already common in parts of Western Europe and the United States (Singleton 2010: 154). The physical culture movement emerged as "a new moral crusade was championing physical vigor" (Albanese 2007: 361). The physical vigor that resulted from exercise was tied to morality, nationalism, and economic vitality since survival in the industrial world was perceived to require physical strength (Singleton 2010: 82–83). Physical culture became increasingly accessible to elite segments of society as various fitness organizations, such as the YMCA (Young Men's Christian Association), flourished.

The valorization of physical fitness traveled from Europe to British India, where Indian yogis assimilated physical culture (Singleton 2010: 81–82). In this way, they salvaged hatha yoga from the onslaughts of Orientalist and reformist criticisms by prescribing it as physical fitness. The result was a "hatha yoga renaissance" (Singleton 2010: 84). Basically, the body practices associated with hatha yoga, that tradition that had been disdained and criticized by European, American, and Indian elites, were now reconstructed in ways that made them salvageable "indigenous" fitness techniques. Singleton suggests that modern yogis began constructing "'indigenous' exercise forms distinct (though often borrowing) from these imported systems...Often, nativized exercise such as this was also referred to as 'yoga'" (Singleton 2010: 82). Indian nationalists often participated in this movement and turned to posture practice as a way to promote "muscular Hinduism," a masculinized ideology incorporating issues of health, strength, and vital energy (Alter 2004: 146; see also Alter 1994). This new form of yoga functioned as a means to physical vigor, which symbolized the power of Indian men in resistance to colonial powers.

The global physical culture had its own countercultural dimensions. Most significantly, it opposed the intellectualism of modern Western European and American culture. Part of the physical culture agenda was to repair the perceived "imbalance of 'body-mind-soul'" because of what was considered too much emphasis on the mind or "intellect" (Singleton 2010: 84).

Simultaneously, however, postural yoga shared certain qualities with yoga systems in which body practices were censored, as prescribed by figures like Vivekananda. First, a spiritual discourse continued to permeate the culture of postural yoga (Singleton 2010: 89–91). In this way, it resembled Vivekananda's raja yoga. It also resembled, however, other systems and organizations constructed out of the global physical culture, such as the YMCA (Singleton 2010: 91). Such organizations as well as postural yoga represented a reawakening of the sacralization of the body (Singleton 2010: 84, 89–94, 119).

It differed, however, from the sacralization of the body by figures like Craddock, Bernard, or Woodroffe. Although they shared with physical culture a desire to counter the mainstream triadic opposition between mind, body, and soul, Craddock, Bernard, and Woodroffe were inspired by tantra to use the body as the locus of erotico-mystical experience and pleasure. Physical culture, on the other hand, provided a context in which physical fitness was perceived to enhance an ascetic and Protestant notion of self-control, moral development, and purity.

Second, modern science was key to the process of constructing postural yoga. Just as Vivekananda argued that the meditational, philosophical, and ethical components of yoga were compatible with science, so those who prescribed postural yoga argued that it could be scientifically proven to improve fitness and health. Joseph S. Alter suggests, through this discourse, "Yoga was modernized, medicalized, and transformed into a system of physical culture" (Alter 2004: 10).

In India, yoga as physical culture underwent growth as demonstrated by the establishment of the first two modern yoga institutions: the Yoga Institute at Santa Cruz, Bombay (established 1918), and the Kaivalyadhama Shrimad Madhava Yoga Mandir Samiti at Lonavla (near Pune) (established 1921). Inspired by Vivekananda's experiential yogic quest for knowledge of the self in combination with the assimilation of physical culture into yoga systems by Indian nationalists, these institutions began disseminating loosely structured, nondogmatic yogic ideas and practices to India's public.[21] Proponents of yoga at these institutes, especially Kaivalyadhama, readily and aggressively appropriated the discourse of science to explain the perceived fitness and health benefits of yoga.

The stretching and muscle-building exercises that became associated with yoga in India were not yet associated with yoga outside of India, but with female physical culture and gymnastics, until widely influential yoga gurus such as Tirumalai Krishnamacharya (1888–1989) and Sivananda Saraswati (1887–1963) connected the two and trained students in postural yoga (Singleton 2010: 154). In fact, Krishnamacharya and Sivananda were the figures most significant in the process of reconstructing yoga in the popular imagination as postural yoga, since some of their students would be responsible for widely disseminating postural yoga within and beyond India.

Training students in the "pan-Indian hub of physical culture revivalism," Mysore, India, from the 1930s to the 1950s, Krishnamacharya constructed an aerobic system of postural yoga whereby the practitioner performed postures in repetition and in sequence (Singleton 2010: 176–177).[22] By the time Krishnamacharya began training a small group of students in the 1930s, yoga in India had come to be associated with the muscle-building and stretching routines that made up physical culture. Krishnamacharya's students, especially B. K. S. Iyengar (b. 1918) and Jois, would successfully market idiosyncratic renditions of postural yoga to a global audience in the second half of the twentieth century.

Sivananda was a yoga guru in Rishikesh who chose to transgress the intimate guru–disciple relationship by participating in the transnational dissemination of his rendition of postural yoga through the distribution of English-language pamphlets throughout India and abroad. Sivananda formalized those activities when he established the Divine

Life Society in 1936.[23] He attracted students from all over the world, including Mircea Eliade, who studied with Sivananda in Rishikesh before becoming one of the most influential twentieth-century scholars of religion.

While Sivananda's appeal to disciples from all over the world made Rishikesh a major hub for postural yoga practice, Krishnamacharya continued to teach students his own rendition of postural yoga in Mysore. Some of his students became yoga teachers themselves, and Iyengar, one of the most famous proponents of yoga in the contemporary world, was one of them. Iyengar lived and studied with this innovative yoga guru in Mysore for three years (1934–1937), after which he moved to Pune, where he eventually became quite popular as a yoga instructor. Iyengar developed his own postural yoga system that was informed by the approach and techniques of his guru as well as increasingly refined biomedical understandings of anatomy and physiology (de Michelis 2004: 197–198).

In the 1920s and 1930s, yogis in India were practicing postural yoga, which developed out of the dialogical exchange between physical culture and modern yoga, but postural yoga was not yet "export ready" (Singleton 2010: 154). In fact, much of the techniques that we today associate with yoga, such as stretching and muscle-building postures, were popular in Europe and the United States by the 1920s but were not yet associated with yoga. Singleton argues, "This supports the hypothesis that postural modern yoga displaced—or was the cultural successor of—the established methods of stretching and relaxing that had already become commonplace in the West" (Singleton 2010: 154). After all, yoga mostly remained associated with the extreme and anti-social among mainstream populations in Western Europe and the United States.

Take Bernard for example. He referred to his own system of yoga as "advanced physical culture," studied many of the trends in the emergent physical culture milieu, and was deeply concerned with the physical fitness of his disciples, yet he remained a countercultural figure. So, despite the assimilations that had taken place between physical culturists and yogis, yoga was generally still associated with social radicals like Bernard in the popular imagination outside of India. In fact, postural yoga would not undergo global popularization until certain social changes enabled postural yoga advocates to flourish in the global fitness market in the second half of the twentieth century.

Conclusion

Perhaps the most important lesson from the early history of modern yoga is that modern yoga is malleable. Yet, with all of the divergences that make up that history, the data reinforce a collective historical pattern: Modern yoga, until the second half of the twentieth century, was countercultural, elite, or scandalous. Before its popularization, modern yoga moved from the counterculture of Indian ascetic renouncers, to the counterculture of turn-of-the-century American practitioners of tantra, to the counterculture of Transcendentalism and metaphysical religion, and to the counterculture of proponents of physical culture. It was not until the late 1960s that it no longer opposed the prevailing cultural norms of Americans and Western Europeans and became readily available to the masses in urban areas across the world. And so all of this begs the question: What changes made that possible?

3

Continuity with Consumer Culture

*Today's Yoga can be adapted to fit all ages, sizes and body
shapes. For the Olympic athlete, a hospital bed, a heated
Yoga studio or seated in a chair—Yoga. Amazing considering Yoga practice probably began 1,000 years ago in a
Himalayan cave!!*

—LILIAS FOLAN (2013)

MODERN YOGA'S EARLY history reaches back to the nineteenth century,
when it developed as a consequence of a series of encounters between
Europeans and Americans interested in topics ranging from metaphysics to fitness and Indian nationalists and reformers interested in promoting yoga as a universal system deemed compatible with modern thought.
In response to various modern commitments, early modern yogis constructed heterogeneous and divergent yoga systems, yet they shared a
desire to reconfigure the relationship between mind, body, and soul in
light of modern science and a concomitant opposition to religious orthodoxies. And it was because of that opposition that, despite the increased
visibility of yoga across the globe, early modern yogis were often marred
in controversy for their countercultural agendas. Modern yoga attracted
small followings made up of those who could afford to be eccentric.

All of that is in stark contrast to modern yoga in the second half of the
twentieth century. In 1961, a Protestant Christian living in a Los Angeles
suburb could choose yoga as a body-maintenance regimen without ever
coming into contact with a yoga guru or joining an elite or countercultural movement. She did not even have to leave her home. She could simply turn on her television and tune in to Richard Hittleman's (1927–1991)
yoga program, *Yoga for Health*.[1] After listening to his convincing argument

that yoga is good for her health, she could choose yoga as one part of her routine of self-development. And soon she would find that many of her neighbors were making the same choice. It was a popular one.

Three developments enabled the global popularization of postural yoga in what had, as a consequence of the dominant socioeconomic forces of market capitalism, become a free market in the second half of the twentieth century. First, the new freedom in physical mobility not only allowed con- ①sumers to travel to other parts of the world and adopt disparate wares, but also allowed business men and women, artisans, and proselytizing teachers to travel outside of their home states or regions to disseminate their wares. Although twentieth-century immigration from India to the United States and Europe had been rare due to legal restrictions, those restrictions were lifted in the 1960s, leading to an influx of immigration, especially to the United States, Britain, and France (Porterfield 2001: 164–65, 203), making consumption across and exchange between Indian, Western European, and North American yoga proponents more possible.

Second, there was widespread disillusionment with established reli- ②gious institutions, and new gurus or *godmen* broke into the competitive spiritual market with wares prescribed as solutions (Swallow 1982: 153; Kakar 1983: 191–192; Fuller 2004 [1992]: 177–181).[2] The transnational rise in adherence to these *entrepreneurial godmen*, as I describe them below, illustrates how yoga proponents assimilated to global socioeconomic developments and constructed religious wares meant for mass consumption.

Participants in the British-American counterculture provide one example of those who were often drawn to religiosities radically distinct from what were perceived as the oppressive, puritanical orthodoxies of the previous generation (Porterfield 2001: 164–65, 203). Many in the counterculture eagerly looked to Indian gurus and their wares, which were perceived to provide pop culture criticism, for religious insights and techniques. Because many countercultural participants, including high-profile ones such as the Beatles, experimented with yoga, yoga became an increasingly visible product desired by many for its perceived ability to improve everyday life as well as, at times, for its soteriological purposes.

Finally, postural yoga increasingly intersected with the emergent global ③consumer culture. In short, while many modern yoga systems, such as Siddha Yoga and Transcendental Meditation, provided pop culture criticism, postural yoga systems generally did not. Rather, they appropriated popular ideas and practices of late-twentieth-century consumer culture. This enabled the shift from increased visibility to popularization, since, in contemporary consumer culture, the masses produce pop culture through consumption (Jameson 1991: 4).

A key factor for the survival of any emergent movement is the need to establish cultural continuity with potential adherents (Stark 1996: 133–146). The most significant site of postural yoga's continuity with potential adherents, primarily urban consumers from middle to upper classes, was the opposition to metanarratives, overarching worldviews believed to have a monopoly on truth. The suspicion of metanarratives in combination with the social and economic processes of globalization, market capitalism, and pluralization had increasingly fragmented consumption in urban areas across the world. More specifically, there increasingly emerged a consumer-oriented approach to worldviews and practices as individuals chose from a variety of such to construct individual *lifestyles*.[3] Postural yoga became one choice among many.

The heterogeneity of the market was key to consumer culture. Technology led to shifts in the division of labor and thus economic institutions. Modernity complicated institutional networks, which had major implications for various areas of life (Berger 1979: 15). Thus an economically privileged person living in London in the 1930s may have been able to choose whether or not to go to a gymnasium to keep physically fit, but a person living there in the 1970s could choose from a variety of fitness institutions, including gymnasiums or yoga, karate, and aerobics studios.[4]

Peter Berger refers to the increased choice that resulted from modernity as "the heretical imperative" (Berger 1979: 28–31). *Heretic* derives from the Greek word *hairetikos*, or "able to choose." Put simply, as a consequence of an increasingly heterogeneous market, consumers by necessity had to make choices. Choosing or "heresy" was no longer simply a possibility, but an imperative (Berger 1979: 28). Berger suggests, "Thus heresy, once the occupation of marginal and eccentric types, has become a much more general condition; indeed, heresy has become universalized" (Berger 1979: 30–31).[5]

Consumer choice ranged from occupation, marriage, leisure activities, and material goods to lifestyle, ideology, and religion. According to Berger:

> In other words, there comes to be a smooth continuity between consumer choices in different areas of life—a preference for this brand of automobile as against another, for this sexual life-style as against another, and finally a decision to settle for a particular

'religious preference'...there is a direct and sociologically analyz-
able link between the institutional and the cognitive transformations brought on by modernity. (Berger 1979: 17)

On the topic of increased choice, Bryan S. Turner adds that consumer choice also became a self-conscious process (1997: 36). In other
words, individuals were aware that their choices reflected individual
preferences.

Although the meanings of goods varied as a consequence of individual
preferences and choices, consumers shared a particular "cultural logic."
The very fact that individuals privileged individual choice is indicative of
a shared culture characterized by a rejection of all-encompassing worldviews and practices.[6] For each consumer, the result was *bricolage*, the
syncretism of heterogeneous ideas and practices constructed by the individual and for the individual (Jameson 1991: 96).

Those things proclaimed to be most sacred to people, including religion, were subject to consumer choice, resulting in "assembled" religious
identities, composed of a bricolage of ideas and practices (Lyon 2000: 76).
One famous study referred to this self-oriented religion as *Sheilahism* after
a nurse who self-consciously constructed her own religion (Bellah et al.
2007 [1985]). Wade Clark Roof suggests that American Baby Boomers
were the first to voluntarily select religious ideas and practices as consumers with a purchasing mentality (Roof and McKinney 1987; Roof 1993;
Roof 1999). Though these studies are skewed toward American subjects,
the observations they provide concerning a consumer-oriented approach
to religion applies to late-twentieth-century urban areas across the world
where the same capitalist socioeconomic developments brought consumer culture to dominance.

The emergent consumer cultural logic included a rejection of any
bifurcation between elite and popular cultures. Whereas strict adherence to modern thought privileged science, technology, and rationalism (the principles of the Enlightenment) and thus maintained an elite
culture believed to be exemplary of these principles, the new consumer
culture featured no such predetermined standards for seeking knowledge or establishing taste (Storey 2009: 183–184).[7] There was no distinction between elite culture and pop culture (Huyssen 1986: viii, 57).[8] The
masses produced pop culture through the act of consumption (Jameson
1991: 4).[9] Thus when a product, such as postural yoga, became widely consumed, it simultaneously became a part of pop culture.

Yoga had never attracted adherents like it did in the second half of the twentieth century. Of course, yoga proponents in different times and places always functioned within markets that featured competition and necessitated assimilation to the demands and desires of potential consumers. And yoga was always context-specific because dominant demands and desires shifted over time and place. But consumer culture provided the context in which yoga could develop into heterogeneous wares that competed in a global market. Modern yoga was no longer the pursuit of a social minority, an elite—not to mention often scandalous—few. It was a part of pop culture and easily accessible. Today it is almost *de rigueur* in urban areas across the world.

In fact, what distinctly marks the second half of the twentieth century as a new phase in modern yoga's history is that yoga became a part of pop culture. Modern yogis no longer engaged—at least not primarily or exclusively—in esoteric, marginal, elite, or countercultural techniques. Rather, proponents engaged in the popular dissemination of yoga as an exoteric body-maintenance regimen for the masses.

Numerous twentieth-century events and individuals were significant portents of postural yoga's popularization. Yoga received positive media attention, and mass-marketed books prescribed yoga as one part of self-development, a popularly valorized goal rooted in the Protestant notion of individual salvation, that could be combined with other worldviews and practices. Indian gurus as well as European and North American yogis began to reconstruct modern yoga systems in ways that universalized them by attributing to them benefits that were removed from specific Indian nationalist and mystical contexts and instead reflected the self-developmental desires that dominated consumer culture. Furthermore, the very method through which people learned yoga changed when, instead of relying on transmission through the traditional intimate guru–disciple relationship usually in the isolated context of an *ashram*, gurus began to market yoga to mass audiences.[10] And finally, with the American and British countercultures, yoga became increasingly transnationally valorized.

Scholars have suggested that we consider modern yoga systems examples of the transplantation of a religious movement from the Indian context to the "Western" one, where they underwent a number of assimilative processes (see, e.g., Caldwell 2001: 25; Williamson 2005: 149; and Williamson 2010).[11] I suggest, however, that these yoga systems did not develop in response to transplantation or as a result of "cultural negotiations" between a static Indian culture and a static Western one. It was, in fact, a movement that developed in response to transnational cultural developments, namely developments in consumer culture.

In this chapter, I seek to understand why it is that nearly all of us who live in urban areas across the world today know someone who "does yoga" as it is colloquially put. And should we choose to do it ourselves, we need not travel farther than a neighborhood strip mall to purchase a yoga mat or attend a yoga class. In short, I seek to understand when and how yoga became a part of pop culture. I will address the rise of consumer culture in an effort to demonstrate that the postural practice we most associate with yoga today underwent global popularization as a consequence of its coincidence with transnational cultural developments. As in Chapter Two, I will not provide an exhaustive history of modern yoga in this period. Rather, my goal is to identify the late-twentieth-century processes that enabled the movement of postural yoga from counterculture to pop culture.

Visibility Without Popularization

What would eventually culminate in the popularization of postural yoga began with increased visibility in places across the world. By the 1930s, many Western Europeans, North Americans, and Indians were aware of postural yoga as a system for attaining physical health—conceptualized in modern terms—but consumers were not yet doing yoga *en masse*. In other words, although there was a steady increase in yoga's visibility, such visibility did not equal popularization.[12] Postural yoga practices were especially rare in the United States and Western Europe. After all, Pierre Bernard's club in Nyack, New York, was the only yoga center in the United States where physical techniques were prominent. And there were no such centers at this time in Europe. Most of those countercultural Americans and Europeans who were practicing yoga were engaged in the meditational and devotional practices prescribed by figures like Paramahansa Yogananda (1893–1952) and Swami Vivekananda.[13] These modern yoga gurus taught renditions of yoga that were radically different from the stretching and muscle-building postural sequences meant to function as fitness routines that we so often associate with yoga today. Some did, however, overlap with postural yoga systems. Yogananda's system, for example, included asana as one component of a complex yogic regimen.

Although by the 1930s postural yoga had become central to Indian physical culture, it remained a part of an elite movement, not a popular one, prescribed by Hindu reformers concerned with emphasizing the scientific components of yoga and Indian nationalists concerned with establishing indigenous opposition to British rule in India. This was not translatable (neither to non-Indian populations nor to much of the Indian populace), and thus it was not yet "export ready."[14]

There was, nevertheless, increased transnational visibility of postural yoga as early as the 1930s, which is particularly evident in some popular English-language publications, such as *Cosmopolitan* and *Time* magazines. Although certain articles provide far more affirmative views of yoga than the many popular English-language publications from the nineteenth and early twentieth centuries (see Chapter Two), they still reflect a tendency to associate yoga with the ideologies and practices of Hindu mystical traditions and not as products available for immediate consumption.

Consider the following examples. A 1935 issue of *Cosmopolitan* included an article with the inviting title, "Yoga for You," by Francis Yeats-Brown (1886–1944), an officer in the British Indian army. The article opens with photographs of Euro-American women in yoga postures and the following lines:

> We've all heard of yoga, the strange philosophy of Hindu mystics—but who'd have thought that the foundation of yoga is—setting-up exercises! Yet can you control your mind if you don't control your body? Here are the first simple steps toward doing both. (Yeats-Brown 1935: 56)

Yeats-Brown explains the physical benefits of yoga along with what he considers its underlying monistic philosophy and mystical aims (Yeats-Brown 1935: 56). He provides some instructions on how to do basic yoga postures but simultaneously insists that yoga must be done in "quiet and regular conditions" and "individual guidance is essential" because yoga can "induce all kinds of physical and psychic disturbances" if performed without the guidance of "a competent instructor" (Yeats-Brown 1935: 182). The article was condensed, syndicated, and redistributed to hundreds of newspapers with the title, "Yoga Is Helpful to Mental, Physical Powers" (Love 2010: 256–257).

In 1941, *Time* magazine published an article titled, "Speaking of Pictures...This is Real Yoga" (Author unknown 1941: 10). This article includes a series of photographs taken at Tirumalai Krishnamacharya's yoga center in Mysore, India. The photographs show the guru's students contorting their bodies into various yoga postures, and the author states, "These pictures present a catalog of 20 of the countless contorted postures by which the soul of an Indian yogi seeks escape from the mortal imprisonment of its human body" (Author unknown 1941: 10).

These articles evidence the increase in global visibility that postural yoga had achieved by the middle of the twentieth century. And both articles, surrounded by advertisements for everything from teeth-cleaning powders to cigars, are quite literally situated within consumer culture. Yet postural yoga itself is not yet a potential product for immediate consumption. Instead it remains a rigorous mystical practice requiring prerequisite Hindu philosophical and metaphysical commitments as well as a commitment to a "competent" teacher or guru. And where was one to find one of those without escaping conventional life for an ashram in India?

Modern Soteriological Yoga

It was not long before many gurus made access to their yoga systems easier by not requiring disciples to come to them in isolated monastic contexts, but instead going out into the world and actively marketing their yoga systems. But many of these earliest widely marketed yoga systems are examples of what I term *modern soteriological yoga* or what Elizabeth de Michelis would categorize as *Modern Denominational Yoga*, not modern postural yoga.[15] These systems, unlike the most widely popularized systems of postural yoga, have emphasized traditional devotion to guru figures and have maintained strict organizational structures and doctrinal commitments.

Though some scholars suggest we consider systems of modern yoga as examples of transplantation of movements from India to Euro-American contexts (e.g., Caldwell 2001: 25; Williamson 2005: 149), many of these yoga systems began to take form long before their diffusion beyond India and remained prominent in India after their diffusion. A closer look at modern soteriological yoga demonstrates that they, like modern postural yoga, developed in response to transnational cultural developments. Furthermore, the successes of the marketing campaigns for soteriological yoga evidence the increase in global visibility of yoga, though these systems were not popularized to the same extent as many systems of postural yoga. For these reasons, a comparison between modern soteriological yoga and modern postural yoga helps illuminate what qualities of postural yoga made its popularization possible. In other words, a comparison of the more limited consumption of soteriological systems relative to postural ones provides insight into how and why some types of yoga underwent popularization. Though many soteriological yoga gurus have functioned to further increase the visibility of yoga since the 1960s by prescribing their yoga systems to large audiences within and beyond India, they have not succeeded in a sustained popularization of those systems.

By the 1960s, urban areas across the world had assimilated to an emergent transnational culture that featured a consumer-oriented approach to worldviews and practices as individuals chose from a variety of such to construct individual lifestyles. *Godmen*, defined by C. J. Fuller as contemporary ascetic guru figures who find fame within and at times beyond India and are revered and worshiped as divine, were in particularly high demand in the global spiritual market (Fuller 2004 [1992]: 177–181). A godman is treated as a literal avatar or "descent" of God.

The late-twentieth-century rise in demand for godmen and sometimes *godwomen* illustrates how devotional traditions adapt to sociological change (Swallow 1982; Kakar 1983; Babb 1987; Gombrich and Obeyesekere 1988; Fuller 2004 [1992]). Some scholars have evaluated how such gurus appealed to contemporary urban middle-class and wealthy individuals who felt threatened by social environments that they no longer controlled in the face of globalization and other modern social processes (Swallow 1982; Kakar 1983: 191–92). They broke into the competitive spiritual market with wares that they prescribed as solutions to the perceived stresses of excess and chaos associated with modern life (Swallow 1982: 153; Kakar 1983: 191–92).[16] They also provided group identity to otherwise uprooted individuals along with a "re-enchantment of the world" or "remystification of the world" through what were believed to be their divinity and miracles (Babb 1987; Gombrich and Obeyesekere 1988). These were entrepreneurial godmen or godwomen who consciously constructed and successfully marketed systems of yoga by associating them with their own personae as well as spiritual wares that were attractive to large target audiences of late-twentieth-century spiritual seekers.

Muktananda (1908–1982) provides an apt example of a late-twentieth-century entrepreneurial godman.[17] Beginning in the 1960s, Muktananda served as the guru of a growing Hindu movement, Siddha Yoga, based on ideas and practices primarily derived from tantra and promising God-realization through the *kripa* or "grace" of the guru. Muktananda constructed and introduced Siddha Yoga in the 1960s and disseminated it to mass audiences in the 1970s and early 1980s. His goal was to bring about a global "meditation revolution" through the diffusion of Siddha Yoga, and he succeeded in attracting thousands of people from urban areas across the world.

Muktananda was believed to be a *siddha* or "perfected one" and therefore equivalent to God. But the conception of God in Siddha Yoga was not one of a distant God, far removed from the reach of his worshippers. In fact, Muktananda was known for his democratic and experiential approach to God—God, according to this guru, was within *everyone*—and the immediate experience of God that the guru allegedly offered. This experience came in the form of *shaktipat diksha* (henceforth *shaktipat*) or "initiation through the descent of *shakti*." Shaktipat is a form of religious initiation through the spontaneous awakening of the previously dormant feminine divine energy believed to reside in all beings (Muller-Ortega 1997: 426–428).[18] In Siddha Yoga, shaktipat is transmitted by the guru to the devotee in an initiatory ritual involving a look, a touch, or Muktananda's initiatory method of choice, a strike on the head with a wand of peacock feathers. Muktananda would deliver shaktipat during "Intensives," choreographed retreats hosted by the guru and his disciples.

Like other Indian godmen and godwomen, Muktananda first responded to the growing demand by marketing himself and his wares to the masses throughout India. In 1960s India, Muktananda lived as a guru more akin to a modern entrepreneurial godman than to a traditional guru.[19] He adopted a godman persona and an exoteric dispensation.

Muktananda introduced Siddha Yoga to disciples at his ashram, Shree Gurudev Ashram (later renamed Gurudev Siddha Peeth), in Ganeshpuri, India. The ashram came to resemble a European- or American-style retreat center more than a traditional, bare ashram and hosted large numbers of disciples from around the world. Disciples visiting or living at the ashram could choose the extent of their commitment to Siddha Yoga. Choices ranged from becoming a fully initiated monastic member of Muktananda's community, where Siddha Yoga functioned as an all-encompassing worldview and system of practice, to incorporating Siddha Yoga into one's spiritual repertoire as one part of an eclectic path toward God- or self-realization. Peter Brent describes the ambiance of Muktananda's ashram:

> The ashram stands in some seventy acres of its own ground. The forecourt is backed by the main building where the offices and the audience hall are. Above and to the left, in a newer building, are the apartment of Swami Muktananda and the women's quarters. Behind this there are gardens, splendid with bougainvilia [sic], and a caged white peacock named Moti. To the left of the first, walled garden is a cluster of buildings and courtyards—the halls where men and women eat, the kitchens, a new guest house still under construction and so on—while in the main garden, mostly scattered about a water tower to the right, stand the chambers and dormitories where male visitors or those permanently on the ashram sleep, their washrooms and lavatories, stone benches for their occasional relaxation. A narrow double door in the back wall of this garden leads to a causeway which divides two patchwork stretches of small paddy fields. Beyond, on a low hill, there stand a cluster of well-appointed bungalows and the marble-lined meditation hall. This last is bare, very still; there is no motion in its air, sounds die within its walls. Its marble floor gleams faintly. A picture of Swami Nityananda dominates it, and others of him line the walls. The hill is quiet, bright with sunshine and bougainvilia [sic]. There are low, spear-leaved guava trees…on the slopes, two or three of the ashram's Westerners work at some improving task—improving for them; it seems to have no value in itself. Outside the bungalows, long chairs stand on the terraces, prepared for the comfortable conversation of the faithful. (Brent 1972: 236)

Though contact with Muktananda still required substantial effort, since disciples had to travel to Ganeshpuri to meet him in the isolated context of the Shree Gurudev Ashram, Muktananda reached out to them by consciously creating a space that would be attractive to and comfortable for a wide range of middle- and upper-class Indian, European, and American disciples. As the Shree Gurudev Ashram Trust, which has administered the financial and legal affairs of the ashram since 1962, accumulated funds, the ashram continued to grow.[20]

Muktananda also reached out to disciples by encouraging an exoteric discourse about the transformative experiences triggered by initiation into Siddha Yoga. He functioned as a model of that discourse by publicly sharing his own experiences. Siddha Yoga was one among many types of yoga available in the spiritual market, so the accessibility of testimonials about its effectiveness could serve to attract disciples as they shopped around and calculated the pros and cons of the various gurus and spiritual wares available to them. The discourse was dominated—and continues to be dominated today—by testimonials of shaktipat, that initiatory ritual that the guru, in this early period of Siddha Yoga's history, delivered to his disciples one at a time.

In the 1970s, Muktananda's active steps toward the mass diffusion of Siddha Yoga expanded to other parts of the world, especially to the United States. As articulated by Muller-Ortega, this move toward making shaktipat readily accessible to a global audience was radical:

> Because of shaktipat's historical rarity and relative unavailability, the notion that Swami Muktananda should have made shaktipat attainable on a wide scale around the world is quite noteworthy. After many centuries of barely being available even in India, its sudden and relatively easy accessibility marks an unprecedented and significant historical shift. It is only when we fathom the rarity of what Swami Muktananda professed to be offering to the world that we can begin to appreciate the boldness and genius of his decision to bring shaktipat out of its millennial obscurity. (Muller-Ortega 1997: 410)

The timing was ideal since immigration restrictions were lifted in the United States and in parts of Europe, and the British-American counterculture was well under way as people increasingly called for a religiosity radically distinct from the orthodoxies of the previous generation. These variables had everything to do with the timing and destinations of Muktananda's world tours, which involved three trips in 1970, from 1974 to 1976, and from 1978 to 1981, to a variety of places, including Italy, Switzerland, France, the United Kingdom, the United States, Australia, and Singapore. The very method through which people learned Siddha Yoga changed when, instead of relying on one-on-one transmission through the traditional guru–disciple relationship in the isolated context of the guru's ashram, Muktananda went out in search of disciples, actively marketing Siddha Yoga, which was now immediately accessible to vast numbers of spiritual seekers. In 1970, he began his mission. By 1974, he was confident that his dissemination would instigate a global "meditation revolution," meaning that Siddha Yoga would survive and even grow long after his death.

Accessibility also increased when Muktananda introduced the Intensive in 1974, making the bestowal of shaktipat available to hundreds of people at a time.[21] Making Siddha Yoga readily accessible in this way was a key step in developing Siddha Yoga as a global movement. To get initiated into Siddha Yoga, all individuals had to do was drop out of conventional life for a couple of days and drop in to an Intensive, hosted in their own city. Unlike the usual modes of initiation in tantric traditions in which disciples often had to permanently renounce conventional forms of life and adopt a systematic program of preparation for initiation into the esoteric core of the tradition, Muktananda's bestowal of shaktipat, the core of Siddha Yoga, was available to the masses for immediate consumption, and, though many individuals did make extensive, long-term commitments to Siddha Yoga, the guru dispensed it independent of the extent of individuals' commitments.

Muktananda remystified the world of his disciples through *shaktipat*, but he also did so through granting them contact, if not always direct contact, with his powerful persona. Muktananda was perceived as the paragon of virtue, the transmitter of power and knowledge, and the "perfected master."[22] Muktananda was considered the perfect model of what all disciples strove to be, especially for monastic disciples, who were expected to be celibate and to perfectly conform to rigorous standards of ethical behavior.

Disciples were drawn to this model of perfection. One disciple actually resorts to gravitational metaphors to describe the disciple's relationship to Muktananda:

> The concept of the relationship between Guru and shishya is that of gravitation, in which the larger body attracts the smaller one. With that gravitational pull, the Guru draws you towards him. When we go a little further, we find that we don't know the nature of this gravitation, how and why it works; we know in what manner gravitation works, but why we do not. (Brent 1972: 237)

Though disciples were drawn to Muktananda, for most of them, direct contact with him was rare, and this was increasingly the case as the movement grew. As we saw above, Muktananda was invested in the growth and stability of Siddha Yoga. Perhaps most importantly, he supported the establishment of Siddha Yoga centers that would provide a sense of group identity to uprooted individuals who could not have regular direct contact with the guru himself. In 1975, Muktananda took a number of additional steps toward making Siddha Yoga accessible, including establishing the Siddha Yoga Dham Associates (SYDA) Foundation, the organization responsible for the financial and organizational structure of Siddha Yoga outside of India. Organizational developments also included the introduction of Siddha Yoga courses and teacher training programs as well as establishing departments for the publication of Siddha Yoga books.[23]

All of this was possible because Muktananda was willing to give selected disciples power in the Siddha Yoga movement. Benton Johnson explains that a founder of a religious movement who facilitates its routinization by giving selected disciples the power to meet the "material needs of the movement" enables its survival (Johnson 1992: S12). Such leaders "are like entrepreneurs with novel products and bold visions who turn out also to be accomplished chief executive officers of an expanding firm" (Johnson 1992: S8). By establishing the SYDA and granting his disciples the power to establish centers where desire for Siddha Yoga could build and spread, Muktananda facilitated the routinization of Siddha Yoga— that is, he facilitated the establishment of a normative structure that met the economic and other practical needs of the movement as a whole. In this way, Muktananda was like other entrepreneurial godmen of his time, such as Maharishi Mahesh Yogi (1918–2008), founder of Transcendental Meditation, who "attended to the long-term advancement of his movement in a calculating manner" (Johnson 1992: S8).

Muktananda marketed Siddha Yoga, which signified a virtuous life, a remystification of the world, and a strong sense of belonging to an organized community. And he made initiation into the Siddha Yoga life readily accessible in the form of shaktipat, conveniently delivered by means of the Intensive. In these ways, Muktananda created for his disciples what Sarah Caldwell, scholar and former Siddha Yoga disciple, describes as "the blissful, perfect, ordered life of utter dependency and spiritual bliss" (Caldwell 2001: 17). Siddha Yoga, unsurprisingly, was in high demand: By the time of Muktananda's death in 1982, Siddha Yoga ashrams and centers had been established in India, the United States, Europe, and Australia.

Other late-twentieth-century entrepreneurial godmen and contemporaries of Muktananda similarly advanced their own nonpostural yoga systems. Maharishi Mahesh Yogi began disseminating his Transcendental

Meditation throughout India and then beyond in 1959 when he traveled to various destinations across the world. Bhaktivedanta Prabhupada (1896–1977) traveled to the United States in 1965 and established the International Society for Krishna Consciousness (ISKCON) in 1966. In 1969, Satya Narayan Goenka (b. 1924) left his home in Myanmar to travel to India with the mission of spreading *vipassana* ("insight meditation" prescribed as a "universal" form of Buddhist meditation). He and his disciples would soon diffuse vipassana beyond India to locations including the United States, Western Europe, and Southeast Asia. They all succeeded, especially Maharishi, in attracting thousands of disciples and living extremely high-profile lives.

As mentioned above, sometimes these figures were *godwomen* (see, e.g., the essays in Pechilis 2004, Chapple 2005, and Raj 2005). Guru Anjali, for example, was a guru from Bengal who established an ashram in 1972 in Long Island, where she taught her interpretation of raja yoga as she believed it was codified in Patanjali's *Yoga Sutras*. Guru Anjali appealed to a variety of American seekers by de-emphasizing many of the Hindu aspects of the yoga tradition, denying any formal affiliations with traditional religious institutions, and, according to Christopher Key Chapple, adapting to the "climate and local flavor of Long Island," inventing "new traditions reflecting life on Long Island" (Chapple 2005: 28). She also avoided using any single name for God. Chapple suggests, "This inclusivist, pluralist approach made her teachings accessible to suburban New York clientele as well as remained true to her own lived pluralism, for she had been married to a Jew for several years" (Chapple 2005: 19). Guru Anjali performed the key roles of a modern guru by facilitating opportunities for disciples "to transcend the constraint of their ego-defined self" and move "beyond the humdrum existence" of consumer life (Chapple 2005: 32).

A Hybrid Case: Preksha Dhyana

While Satya Narayan Goenka's vipassana, Maharishi's Transcendental Meditation, Prabhupada's ISKCON, Guru Anjali's raja yoga, and Muktananda's Siddha Yoga all became increasingly popular within and beyond India in the 1970s, a modern variety of Jain meditation and yoga, *preksha dhyana*, emerged. Mahaprajna (introduced in the Preface), the *acharya* (monastic leader) of the Jain Shvetambara Terapanth, introduced preksha dhyana, a hybrid of modern soteriological and modern postural yoga, and sought to diffuse it within and beyond India. Preksha dhyana was a Terapanth Jain attempt to join the newly emerging competitive yoga market where yoga had become a transnational product for improving everyday life and sometimes for soteriological aims.[24]

To understand the extent to which the introduction of preksha dhyana was radical from the perspective of traditional Jain thought and especially traditional Terapanth thought, one must consider the history of the sect. Bhikshu (1726–1803), the founder and first acharya of the Jain Terapanth in Rajasthan, maintained that the Jain commitment to *ahimsa* or "nonviolence" is about the purification of the soul in its quest toward release from the body. Bhikshu was a Shvetambara reformer who left his order in 1759, arguing that the Jain monastic path had moved away from the original teachings of Mahavira, the historical founder of the Jain tradition. He argued that authentic ascetic behavior included wearing the *muhpatti* or "mouth-shield," rejecting image worship, and observing elaborate fasting.[25] Bhikshu also insisted that the total authority of a single acharya was a necessary part of the reformation process in order to prevent schisms or laxity in monastic behavior. He established a new order in 1760 and called it the Terapanth, asserting that it returned to Mahavira's dualist ontology, which deems the material world to be inherently violent and has its logical end in ascetic religious practice that involves the reduction and eventual elimination of all physical and social action.[26]

Today the Terapanth continues to function as a Shvetambara Jain sect that, in contrast to most other Jain sects, is a proselytizing organization.[27] Its current status is the culmination of numerous innovations during the acharyaship of the ninth acharya, Tulsi (1914–1997), between 1936 and 1994. Tulsi led an ecumenical campaign for global peace in response to what he deemed to be a violent world plagued by modernity. Beginning around 1943, while World War II raged on, Tulsi showed concern over the dreadful state of global affairs and began a quest to increase his social engagement (Tulsiramji Maharaj 1945: 3). Basically, he responded to what he considered the "universal unrest" caused by the war but also by what he perceived to be the rise in moral problems due to processes of industrialization, urbanization, and materialism, all of which he associated with modernity (Tulsiramji Maharaj 1945: 3). Tulsi suggested that the Jain path was a universal solution, referring to Mahavira's teaching on nonviolence as a "World Religion" (Tulsiramji Maharaj 1945: 6; Vishrutavibha 2007: 29–30). All of this occurred despite the Terapanth position that monastics should not engage in worldly action, that they should withdraw from society and from what Tulsi himself called the "vomit" of worldly affairs (Vallely 2002: 39).

On March 2, 1949, Tulsi founded the Anuvrat or "Lesser Vows" movement dedicated to "taking Jainism beyond the Jains."[28] The lesser vows
are qualified versions of the five Jain *mahavratas* or "great vows": ahimsa
(nonviolence), *satya* (truth-telling), *asteya* (nonstealing), *brahmacharya*
(celibacy), and *aparigraha* (nonattachment).[29] The Anuvrat movement
prescribed the lesser vows for all laypeople, Jain and non-Jain. The movement dramatically shifted the public face of the Terapanth in India from
its status as an especially ascetic body-denying, society-denying, and
world-denying Jain sect to what resembled a social movement.

When one of Tulsi's wealthy disciples donated sixty acres of land in
the town of Ladnun in the Nagaur district of Rajasthan to establish a Jain
learning center, Tulsi responded in 1970 with the establishment of Jain
Vishva Bharati (JVB), a global organization for disseminating Terapanth
ideology and practice while adapting the sect to changes in the modern
world. The Terapanth constructed the first JVB center in Ladnun, and it
was there that one of Tulsi's closest disciples, the monk Muni Nathmal
(1920–2010), played a vital role in yet another Terapanth innovation.[30]

Nathmal received permission from Tulsi to take leave from his regular monastic duties in order to study ancient Jain scriptures in search
of a "lost" form of Jain yoga.[31] In 1975, Nathmal introduced preksha
dhyana—literally "concentration of perception," but translated by insiders to the tradition as "insight meditation and yoga." He suggested that
preksha dhyana was a universal system that had been lost and was now
rediscovered, that it was grounded in science, and that his rediscovery
depended primarily on his experiences through personal experimentation.[32] Tulsi honored Nathmal by giving him a new name, Mahaprajna or
"Great Wisdom." Mahaprajna was initiated as the tenth acharya in 1994
and continued in that role until his death on May 9, 2010.

On the one hand, the introduction of preksha dhyana was not particularly innovative because it was consistent with other trends that many
Rajasthanis would have been familiar with in the 1970s, namely that
modern systems of both soteriological and postural yoga were increasingly diffused within and beyond India. On the other hand, preksha dhyana was a radical innovation because, in contrast to the body-denying,
society-denying, world-denying Jain ascetic ideal, preksha dhyana
included modern systems of diet and physical exercise in the form of postures aimed at worldly goals, namely health. Furthermore, Mahaprajna's
construction of preksha dhyana demonstrated the phenomenon whereby
postural yoga, by appropriating the physiological and anatomical discourse

of biomedicine, somaticizes a system that was traditionally a metaphysical practice oriented around the manipulation of subtle energies.

The Terapanth acharya required all monastics to practice preksha dhyana and prescribed it for all lay followers of the Anuvrat program for self-improvement. This led to an additional innovation, since representatives were needed to teach preksha dhyana throughout India and the world. Thus, beginning in 1980, the Terapanth introduced the *saman* order of intermediary monastic renunciates who are not fully initiated into the monastic order.[33] Although in 1986 four *samanas* or male saman were initiated, the large majority were and remain *samanis* or female saman.[34]

What makes this order particularly innovative is the fact that the rules governing the saman monastic lifestyle are more lax than those for fully initiated monastics. The saman are allowed to travel by means of mechanical transportation, live in buildings constructed or purchased especially for them, not wear the mouth-shield, and establish long-lasting relationships with the laity.[35] This enables them to travel throughout India and abroad to diffuse preksha dhyana. Such an innovation was radical for a Jain sect founded in 1760 on a call for reformation, defined by Bhikshu in terms of returning the Jain tradition to the ascetic path of purification.

Tulsi and Mahaprajna saw the changes as both innovations and reformations. They were reformations insofar as they were considered consistent with the teachings of Mahavira and his instructions to preach Jain doctrine and practice to all living beings, but they were innovations insofar as they adapted to advancements in modern technology and globalization.[36]

Preksha dhyana's dissemination has two dimensions. First, in his explication for the monastic or advanced adept, Mahaprajna appropriated metaphysical conceptions from hatha yoga with regard to the manipulation of the subtle body for the sake of increasing knowledge of the transcendent self.[37] In this way, he constructed preksha dhyana as part of the ascetic soteriological path of the monastic. In his written work on preksha dhyana, Mahaprajna moves back and forth rather abruptly between an ascetic system of bodywork and a de-asceticized affirmation of the body as a tool for self-discovery. As an ascetic system for Jain monastics and advanced adepts, preksha dhyana serves to purify the self from the body and to bring about the experience of the self. In this context, it bears a strong resemblance to hatha yoga, which has historically emphasized esoteric mysticism and often utilizes the body as the locus of mystical experience (see Chapter One). Mahaprajna's description of subtle anatomy closely resembles that of hatha yoga (Mahaprajna 2003b: 23). He even makes explicit references to kundalini yoga, called *antaryatra* or the "internal trip" in the preksha dhyana system (Mahaprajna 2003b: 21).[38] Here a meditational program is central to preksha dhyana. It does not involve posture except for the preliminary adoption of an appropriate meditative posture, though a variety of stretching and muscle-building exercises that are popular in the postural yoga world, such as the *surya namaskar* (sun salutation) postural sequence, as well as individual postures, such as *bhujanga asana* (cobra posture), *sarvanga asana* (shoulder-stand posture), and *chakra asana* (wheel posture), are accepted as preliminary steps because increased bodily flexibility and strength are believed to contribute to the practitioner's ability to meditate comfortably, without bodily distractions, for long periods of time.[39]

Though postural exercises are preliminary to the central meditative program for monastics and other advanced adepts, Mahaprajna prescribed them for everybody as a solution to what he deemed illnesses of modernity and especially urban lifestyles linked to a diet of unhealthy nonvegetarian foods, lack of exercise, overconsumption, and increased stress. Mahaprajna associated each yoga posture with certain physiological benefits with regard to basic aches and pains, and cures of chronic illnesses such as heart disease and diabetes. He also associated each part of the subtle body with a physiological component. The endocrine system played a particularly key role. Mahaprajna suggested that the manipulation of subtle energies in the body brings about shifts in the release of chemicals and hormones in the body, which in turn positively affect both mental and physical health (see, e.g., Mahaprajna 2009: 11, 75).[40]

Despite biomedical discourse, a distinctly Jain soteriology remains, and thus improving the body is a means, not an end in itself. In this way, Mahaprajna echoes Vivekananda (introduced in Chapter Two), who suggested that the physical benefits of yoga were inferior to what he considered the true aim of yoga: spiritual development (Vivekananda 1992 [1896]: 20). According to Mahaprajna, the healthy body is a means for perceiving one's self, which lies buried within the body, beneath layers upon layers of gross body and subtle body (Mahaprajna 2004: 27). Preksha dhyana could make the digging through such layers possible; this is why it is often referred to as "insight" meditation. Mahaprajna thus maintained a traditional Jain body-negating soteriology but qualified the concomitant ascetic ideal in the everyday body maintenance of the practitioner, where the body's health is embraced as a legitimate, if preliminary, aim.

Mahaprajna suggested that it is necessary to achieve bodily health in order to more easily perceive dualist reality. He claimed that by permanently changing the body hormonally, preksha dhyana functions to improve one's spiritual state by getting rid of "psychological distortions" or negative emotions such as hate, cruelty, and fear, which he believed result from an imbalanced and unregulated endocrine system and which prevent purification from karma (Mahaprajna 2004: 85). According to Mahaprajna, most diseases are products of psychosomatic processes. Thus, insofar as one practices preksha dhyana, the "physiotherapy" for controlling hormonal secretions, one reduces negative emotions that function as obstacles to both good health and a better spiritual state.[41] The advanced adept can then more easily perceive the distinction between the body and the self and thus progresses toward the Jain soteriological goal: the realization of the true self and subsequent release of the self from the body.

In the second dimension of preksha dhyana's dissemination, Mahaprajna joined numerous entrepreneurial godmen who constructed new yoga systems meant for large target audiences of late-twentieth-century seekers. This second dimension is particularly visible in the yoga classes at the JVB centers, where the central and marginal dimensions of preksha dhyana are reversed. In the frequently offered yoga classes, the samanis focus primarily on modern yoga postures, and the central aspects of the meditational program are largely ignored. Although they do incorporate certain meditational practices, including mantra and relaxation, they do so minimally, usually for only a few moments at the beginning or end of class. Sometimes the samanis offer separate classes that focus not on physical exercise, but on meditation. They also offer camps in which practitioners remove themselves from the stresses of everyday life for a few days during which they learn the complete meditational program of preksha dhyana. The samanis, however, describe how very few students come when a meditation class is offered, but several more come for yoga classes that emphasize physical exercises.[42]

In such classes, the samanis address their students' body aches or chronic health issues. This reflects their students' concerns with enhancing their everyday life through yoga. Primarily, students mention health and fitness as the reasons they practice yoga.[43] In addition, students often express a desire to reduce stress, improve their physical appearance, and possibly, along the way, "achieve something spiritual."[44] Few students voice an interest in yoga as a means to advanced progress along the Jain path to salvation.[45] In response to their students' interests and concerns, the samanis' teachings differ from those found in the monastic context, meditation classes, and camps for soteriologically oriented lay practitioners insofar as the focus is not on ascetic body and meditative work for the sake of the purification and perception of the self, but on body maintenance and the enhancement of life according to modern ideas about fitness, beauty, and health. For most lay practitioners, the healthy body is not a preliminary but rather a final goal.

The samanis maintain Mahaprajna's assertion that yoga's health-enhancing techniques are simply means to a soteriological aim.[46] Yet, as a practical response to most people's exclusive concern with health, the samanis often focus on the health benefits of yoga postures in the context of their global diffusion of preksha dhyana. The samanis must market preksha dhyana according to the desires and needs prevalent in the global yoga market. This is in line with the fact that the introduction of this new monastic order was a self-conscious attempt to establish continuity with the dominant late-twentieth-century global culture.

Since the introduction of their order in 1980, samanis have established four major JVB centers outside of India, in London, the United Kingdom; Houston, Texas; Iselin, New Jersey; and Orlando, Florida. At each of these centers, they repeat their late guru's proclamation that preksha dhyana is a tool for achieving health. Yet, like their guru, they demonstrate a flux between, on the one hand, commitments to a Jain dualist ontology and a concomitant ascetic soteriology, and on the other hand an affirmation of bodily aims as legitimate goals in the context of their postural yoga classes.

In addition to attracting yoga practitioners to preksha dhyana by providing postural yoga classes, the samanis have also served to attract devotees to the Terapanth acharyas as mediators to them. Both Tulsi and Mahaprajna served as godmen. Both gurus were regarded as having characteristically auspicious bodies, particularly because of their elongated ears, which are considered a sign of advanced spiritual power in traditional South Asian religious culture. Miracles were also attributed to them. Disciples are especially apt to tell stories of Tulsi and Mahaprajna's paranormal abilities to communicate with them at long distances.[47]

Chhogmal Choprha, a Terapanth author writing during Tulsi's term as acharya, provides the following description of the Terapanth view of the acharya:

He is the Supreme Head of the Order and all Sadhus and Sadhwis owe allegiance to Him and obey His commands and follow His instructions. He is the highest spiritual authority and all [monastics and lay people] pay their unstinted homage to Him (*sic*) He is the highest living deity—the object of the greatest reverence of all followers, laymen or Sadhus. He is the brightest Moon round whom the entire system of stars move. He is the Heart and Soul of the entire...*Jain Swetamber Terapanth Sect*. He is the greatest Administrator of law and discipline, the commander-in-chief under whom moves the whole noble band of warriors for the emancipation of soul. (Choprha n.d.: 12)

Tulsi and Mahaprajna's circles of disciples were made up, in large part, of self-identifying Terapanths in Rajasthan who were most often members of the same caste as Bhikshu, the Bisa Osval merchant caste, and remained ethnically Rajasthani, although they attributed universal applicability and accessibility to their gurus' teachings. But self-identifying Terapanths were not their only disciples. There were also devotional communities in Indian urban centers who were far more diverse and were made up of middle- to upper-class urban Jains and Hindus from various sectarian traditions. Finally, there were Jains and Hindus in diaspora.

Mahaprajna's success in attracting so many disciples can be attributed to his godman persona. For that persona he received much publicity. In June 2009, while in Ladnun, thousands of Hindus and Jains from all over the country traveled to Ladnun to see him and perhaps to gain just a few minutes of direct access to him in celebration of his birthday.[48] In Jaipur, the closest major urban area to Ladnun, Mahaprajna's popularity was widespread throughout the city. The urban middle class in Jaipur, both Jain and non-Jain, were familiar with Mahaprajna and his late guru, Tulsi, and consistently affirmed their spiritual qualities, especially those of Mahaprajna. They claimed that he was a "great guru" with regard to spirituality and health.[49]

Mahaprajna was also well known in Jain diaspora communities. In Houston, Texas, for example, Jains from various sectarian traditions revered Mahaprajna as a spiritual and health guru. In October 2009, Samani Akshaya Pragya and Samani Vinay Pragya opened the largest JVB center outside of India, the JVB Houston Preksha Meditation Center, to accommodate these disciples. Although samanis ran and managed the center, they claimed that, like the other JVB centers, it was nonsectarian.[50]

Yet pictures of Mahaprajna adorn the walls, and disciples there affirm that
Mahaprajna was not a guru to Terapanths alone. Almost all of the attendees at the Terapanth-run centers in the United States and Britain are members of the Indian diaspora, most of whom self-identify as non-Terapanth
Jain and often Hindu, and all of them show reverence for the samanis as
representatives of the "great guru," Mahaprajna.

Tulsi and Mahaprajna both received attention from thousands of disciples following the introduction of the Anuvrat movement, and preksha
dhyana required innovations if the Terapanth was to remain committed
to the Jain ascetic ideal, especially since the new agenda included the dissemination of preksha dhyana outside of India. Whereas the Terapanth
never entirely resolved this problem, it made an important attempt with
the introduction of the samani order. The Terapanth's inability to entirely
resolve the tension was evidenced in the persistent steps to negotiate the
relationship between Mahaprajna and his disciples. For example, in June
2009, Mahaprajna announced steps to further distance himself from disciples by means of new prohibitions controlling devotional boundaries.
These announcements came on his ninetieth birthday and functioned
as part of his attempt to retreat from social action into solitude in preparation for death.[51] First, he claimed every Tuesday as a day of solitude,
when he would not interact with anyone outside of his immediate circle
of monks. Every day, busloads of people would arrive in Ladnun from
all over the world. They were filled with people who traveled hours (and
sometimes days) in order to have just a few minutes with the guru. Now,
at least one day a week would be for him to focus on his own spiritual
practice rather than on those who desperately desired his guidance.
Second, he implemented a new rule preventing all laypeople from touch-
ing his feet, a traditional South Asian sign of reverence. This evidenced
his attempt to further withdraw from the world as he neared death, since
that withdrawal served to increasingly prevent the accumulation of additional karmic matter. When people touched his feet, the physical contact
was believed to distribute some of their karmic matter to him.

By means of their intermediary status, the samanis could absorb much
of the karmic matter that otherwise would be brought upon Mahaprajna
through interaction with disciples. The samanis partook in most interactions for him, not just in Ladnun, but also in every other place they
traveled or established JVB centers for the sake of diffusing preksha dhyana. Nevertheless, photographs of Mahaprajna were found in every JVB
center where the samanis taught, and the samanis regularly reminded

students of Mahaprajna's supremecy, thus maintaining the concentration of authority in the person of the guru.

Postural Yoga Gurus Become Mass Marketers

The successes of modern soteriological yoga systems testify to the increased visibility and consumption of yoga in the late twentieth century, especially in the 1960s and 1970s, in areas across the globe. Even Jains introduced a modern yoga system despite the fact that some of its aims dramatically differed from those of the traditional Jain soteriological path. The entrepreneurial spirit that characterized the consumer culture landscape influenced advocates of modern soteriological yoga, especially insofar as spiritual seekers were encouraged to combine yoga with previously held beliefs or practices according to individual preferences. The entrepreneurial spirit, however, was strongest among yoga proponents concerned exclusively with postural yoga. It was those proponents who established the greatest continuity with the growing global consumer culture.

Long-term commitment to soteriological yoga systems frequently required adherents to learn Sanskrit or other Indian languages in order to systematically study large bodies of sacred literature and to patiently maintain a committed relationship in an inferior position vis-à-vis a qualified guru for years. Furthermore, the fact that entrepreneurial godmen required serious adherents to privilege particular worldviews over others, despite their claims to universalism or nonsectarianism, made them less successful in the global yoga market than the thoroughly individualistic varieties of postural yoga. Especially Maharishi, Prabhupada, and Mahaprajna's rejection of an entirely consumer-oriented approach to religious and body practices in favor of particularized philosophical and devotional commitments situated them in the folds of Hindu or Jain traditions.[52]

And sometimes they were situated in esoteric traditions. For example, Muktananda's end-of-life choice to embrace certain transgressive tantric dimensions of yoga that were not previously a part of his public persona contributed to the decline in Siddha Yoga's success.[53] There were accusations of improprieties against Muktananda following his death— Muktananda was accused of having sex with young female disciples, including some teenagers as a part of esoteric rituals (see Caldwell 2001; Urban 2003: 243–250; Jain 2014b: 203–207).[54] Furthermore, soteriological yoga systems ultimately privileged such aims as God-realization or self-realization over the common everyday aims of the masses. Proponents of ISKCON, for example, shared a view of the current age of time as particularly degraded largely due to materialism, scientific technology, and consumerism (Gelberg 1989: 138; Saliba 1989: 227). According to Steven J. Gelberg, "The devotee sees the whole modern world, one might say, as an unpleasant intrusion into sacred time and space" (Gelberg 1989: 138). ISKCON, therefore, offered an alternative, "antimaterialistic lifestyle" (Saliba 1989: 227). All of this was neither feasible nor desirable for the vast majority of cosmopolitan consumers. In short, in their rejection of an overwhelmingly consumer-oriented approach to religious wares and in their devotional, philosophical, or esoteric underpinnings, soteriological yoga systems required serious adherents to drop out of conventional life to a degree that postural yoga systems did not.

The abundant successes of postural yoga systems stemmed from their proponents' willingness to consistently make concessions to consumer cultural norms and to drop traditional requirements of yoga study and practice. As Elizabeth de Michelis points out, postural yoga's popularization is explained in part by the fact that it provided direct access to the perceived benefits of yoga, rather than indirect access through the intermediary role of a teacher or text (2004: 250). Increasingly, yoga gurus did not require disciples to drop out of the conventional world— to no greater extent than for a thirty- or sixty-minute yoga class and, in many cases, to an even lesser extent—in order to learn and do yoga. Instead, their marketing campaigns attempted to convince people to choose their particular renditions of yoga as one part of individual programs of self-development that could be combined with other aspects of one's life. Their various renditions of yoga were compatible with the underlying logic of consumer culture. They marketed forms of yoga that did not privilege any religious, ethnic, or national metanarrative, replacing those forms with ones that facilitated individual choice. More specifically, many of them marketed postural yoga systems that were less explicitly (if at all) associated with either religious mystical traditions or Indian nationalism. All of this amounted to them responding to a transnational market in which wares were most successful when they could be easily fit into individualized lifestyles. Consequently, many postural yoga gurus, such as B. K. S. Iyengar, Bikram Choudhury (b. 1946), and John Friend (b. 1959), abandoned all or many of the rules, such as those dealing with alms, celibacy, scriptural study, and retreat from society or social norms that traditionally functioned to separate the yoga practitioner from society so that they could mass market a form of yoga that functioned as fitness, something increasingly valorized in urban areas around the world as the twentieth century progressed.

There were many key players in the early global dissemination of postural yoga. For example, in India, the first modern yoga institutions, the Yoga Institute at Santa Cruz, Bombay (established 1918) and the Kaivalyadhama Shrimad Madhava Yoga Mandir Samiti at Lonavla (established 1921), both introduced in Chapter Two, prescribed yoga systems believed to be uniquely Indian forms of physical culture that were compatible with modern science and available to anyone regardless of religious or institutional commitments. Disciples of Vivekananda founded both institutes, and thus their teachings reflected Vivekananda's understanding of yoga as "body-mind-spirit training" (de Michelis 2004: 189). In other words, although their concern was not exclusively with postural yoga, physical practice was prescribed as one part of a larger yoga system.

Many advocates of postural yoga not only maintained a universalized vision of yoga, but also actively delivered it around the world. Selvarajan Yesudian (1916–1998) was one of the first Indian yogis to mass-market postural yoga beyond India. Born in Madras, Yesudian traveled to Europe in 1936 to study medicine. He met the Hungarian spiritual teacher and mystic Elisabeth Haich (1897–1994), and together they wrote what would become the widely successful Hungarian-language publication *Sport és Jóga* (*Sport and Yoga*) (1941). The book featured photographs of the exceedingly fit Yesudian performing postures, breathing exercises, and meditation. It sold so many copies that it was translated into several different languages, including German in 1949 and English as *Yoga and Health* in 1953. Together, Yesudian and Haich also opened yoga schools in Zurich and Ponte Tresa, Switzerland. Both schools remained open until 1989.

In Rishikesh, Sivananda, also introduced in Chapter Two, taught a rendition of postural yoga that aimed toward enhancing the mind and body according to modern biomedical conceptions of health. Sivananda's appeal to disciples from all over the world made Rishikesh a major hub for postural yoga practice. Yoga was an easy and universally accessible practice, according to Sivananda, that did not require one to forfeit any ethnic, philosophical, or religious commitments. Yoga, according to Sivananda, was meant for anybody interested in enhancing the body and mind through physical exercise. Sivananda's universalization of yoga reached its culmination in 1959 with his English-language book, *Yogic Home Exercises: Easy Course of Physical Culture for Modern Men and Women.*

One of Sivananda's students from Germany, Boris Sacharow (1899–1959), having never actually traveled to Rishikesh, became a disciple through the guru's English-language pamphlets. In 1947, Sivananda gave him the title *yogiraj* or "master of yoga" (Strauss 2005: 41).[55] With this honorary title serving to legitimize his expertise on yoga, Sacharow opened the first yoga school in Germany (Strauss 2005: 41–42). Another one of Sivananda's students, Vishnudevananda (1927–1993), established International Sivananda Yoga Vedanta centers and ashrams in locations around the world as well as the Sivananda Yoga Teachers' Training Course, which serves to regulate Sivananda Yoga to this day.

Krishnamacharya, another postural yogi introduced in Chapter Two, continued to teach students his own rendition of postural yoga in Mysore. Some of his students became postural yoga entrepreneurs, delivering postural yoga to consumers beyond India. Indra Devi (1899–2002), Krishnamacharya's only female student, moved to the United States after studying in Mysore. She was originally from Riga, Latvia (formerly Livonia), but chose to live and teach yoga in Hollywood, California, where her clientele included celebrities such as Marilyn Monroe and Gloria Swanson. Devi opened her first yoga studio in 1947, where she taught yoga as a form of physical fitness that could be incorporated into various programs of self-development.

Iyengar, one of the most famous proponents of yoga in the contemporary world, was another entrepreneurial postural yogi who had studied under Krishnamacharya. Iyengar lived and studied with this innovative yoga guru in Mysore for three years (1934–1937), after which he moved to Pune, where he eventually became quite popular as a yoga instructor. Iyengar's postural yoga system attracted a number of wealthy and influential celebrities, including the famous violinist Yehudi Menuhin (1916–1999) in 1952. With celebrities' patronage, in the 1950s, he traveled to London, Switzerland, the United States, and Paris to teach postural yoga. By Iyengar's third trip to London in 1960, he had established a permanent group of students. From this point on, he would return every year to teach them.

By 1960, postural yoga was a product that people across the world were choosing as part of their everyday body-maintenance regimens. By means of the popular dissemination of postural yoga in large part because of

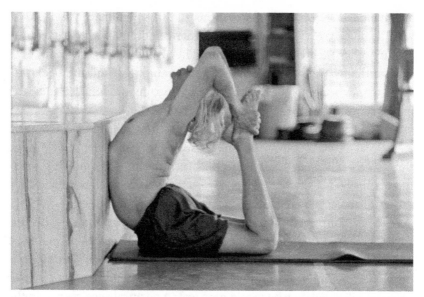

FIGURE 3.1 B. K. S. Iyengar practicing *kapota asana* or "pigeon posture" at the age of 91. Photographed by Jake Clennell. (Courtesy of Jake Clennell.)

[handwritten marginalia: how and what is detachable in yoga?]

the above-listed key figures, postural yoga became something that was increasingly prescribed and consumed as a product independent of ethnic, philosophical, or religious identities or commitments. Postural yoga was instead a product that could be chosen as a body-enhancing practice that was one part of individual regimens of self-development, and it was being packaged in this way for transnational audiences.

Iyengar Yoga was particularly successful (Fig. 3.1). Iyengar prescribed a thoroughly individualistic system of postural yoga that was a rigorous and disciplined form of body maintenance that required the use of fitness tools, such as belts, bricks, and ropes. He published his *Light on Yoga* in 1966, and it instantly became the global standard reference on modern yoga as a body practice (de Michelis 2004: 198.). The text became, according to de Michelis, "the acknowledged point of reference in the sense that no modern postural yoga practitioner or school could afford to ignore its existence" (de Michelis 2004: 211). Although postural yogis already had three reference works on yoga postures—Yesudian and Haich's *Sport és Jóga* (1941), also published in English as *Yoga and Health* (1953), Theos Bernard's *Hatha Yoga* (1944), and Vishnudevananda's *The Complete Illustrated Book of Yoga* (Vishnudevananda 1960)—Iyengar's book was particularly attractive to a consumer culture audience insofar as it included step-by-step instructions so that individuals could choose yoga as one part of their self-development regimen without having to give up other lifestyle commitments. They could do yoga without even leaving their homes. Furthermore, in meticulous detail, the book provided biomedical explanations of each posture and its fitness and health benefits.

In the late 1960s, a mass market for postural yoga classes emerged. Iyengar Yoga classes even became available at American YMCAs and through the Clapton Adult Education Institute in London. This was a thoroughly body-centered variety of yoga that was deemed beneficial for a variety of consumers regardless of various other commitments.

Furthermore, even though Sivananda died in 1963, many of his disciples succeeded in popularizing body-centered yoga in this period. Most significantly, Chidananda Sarasvati (1916–2008) traveled throughout the world teaching postural yoga and attracting disciples.[56] His disciples included Lilias Folan, who would propagate a postural yoga system in the 1970s on American television. Yet, before Folan began her popularization of postural yoga, Hittleman's *Yoga for Health* had become syndicated on various television stations all over the United States by 1970, and by 1971, it was shown on British television. Eleven years after Hittleman's 1961 debut of *Yoga for Health*, in 1972 Folan debuted *Lilias, Yoga, and You!* The show first aired on Cincinnati's PBS station, but within the year it was on PBS stations across the United States. It continued to air until 1992. The biggest challenge, according to Folan, "was convincing Public Television that yoga wasn't peculiar, strange and un-American, that it *isn't* a religion—that was the big one" (quoted in Syman 2010: 247). The rendition of modern yoga that Folan propagated on television, like that of Iyengar, was a thoroughly individualistic postural yoga system. It was about self-development through enhancing physical fitness and health, and anyone could choose it regardless of religious, ethnic, or national identity.

Conclusion

To understand how modern yoga underwent popularization, one must understand consumer culture. Yoga entered a new phase of development in the context of consumer culture beginning in the second half of the twentieth century. In consumer culture, modern yoga was no longer a countercultural or elite movement but was a part of transnational pop culture. Popularization did not happen equally everywhere. Especially in more conservative sectors of North American and Western European cultures, residual cultural norms that opposed experimentation with anything deemed to have non-Christian origins prevented the popularization of yoga. Texas yoga practitioner, teacher, and studio owner Roger Rippy, for example, described growing up in Fort Worth, Texas, where doing yoga "could quite possibly have gotten you beaten up" (Yoga One 2013). Yet in many urban areas across the globe, postural yoga was becoming increasingly accessible and commonly practiced among the general populace as its proponents established cultural continuity with consumer culture.

The adaptation of modern yoga to consumer culture reflects a response to transnational developments in consumer culture, not a transplantation of a bounded system from one static culture to another. Here Hugh B. Urban's discussion of Osho-Rajneesh, a modern tantric guru known for his voracious appetite for sex and money, is relevant (Urban 2005). Urban corrects the vision of modern tantra as a result of the "Europeanization" or "Americanization" of religion and suggests:

> Rather, the real threat today is the spread of consumer capitalism and the domination of the global marketplace over all local economies, polities, and cultural forms—a process that is no longer dominated by the West, no longer a matter of either "occidentalization" or "orientalization," but a far more complex product of transnational capitalism." (Urban 2005: 187)

Although many systems of modern yoga that did not concede to consumer trends were diffused throughout the world, including Hindu, Buddhist, and even Jain varieties, the most successful attempts at diffusion occurred when proponents consistently *did* concede to consumer cultural trends. These were most often the postural yoga proponents.

Their popularization of postural yoga reflects a phenomenon in the history of religions as a whole in which individuals and institutions continuously construct and reconstruct their wares anew in response to new social, cultural, and historical contexts. Thus, whether or not we respond pessimistically or disapprovingly to transnational consumer culture wiping out cultural difference, the fact remains that yoga's changes in light of its shifting contexts are just examples of a more general human phenomenon. Despite the fact that postural yoga reflects that general phenomenon, there are a number of unique qualities of postural yoga that resulted from its adaptation to the specific context of consumer culture, and I now turn to a more detailed analysis of those qualities.

4

Branding Yoga

[People know about physically oriented yoga] but as we grow they are going to learn about Anusara. Then people can choose—either they are going to go to a fast-food joint or a fine restaurant.

—JOHN FRIEND (2010)

IN THE 1980s, 1990s, and 2000s, the postural yoga market became increasingly diversified and came to feature endless yoga brands constructed and marketed for immediate consumption. Proponents of postural yoga brands took a variety of steps toward building what would become successfully marketed yoga products. Consider John Friend.[1] In October 1989, long-time yoga student and white American suburbanite Friend traveled to India to study with yoga masters. First, he went to Pune for a one-month intensive postural yoga program at the Ramamani Iyengar Memorial Yoga Institute, founded by world-famous yoga proponent B. K. S. Iyengar, who was introduced in preceding chapters. Following Friend's training in Iyengar Yoga, he traveled to the Gurudev Siddha Peeth ashram in Ganeshpuri, India, where he met Gurumayi Chidvilasananda (b. 1954), the current guru of Siddha Yoga and disciple of Muktananda, who was introduced in Chapter Three.

Friend spent the next seven years deepening his understanding of both Iyengar Yoga and Siddha Yoga. He earned two Iyengar Yoga teaching certificates and taught Iyengar Yoga in Houston, Texas. Every summer, he traveled to Siddha Yoga's Shree Muktananda Ashram in upstate New York, where he would study for one to three months at a time.

Friend founded his own postural yoga system, Anusara Yoga, in 1997 in The Woodlands, a Houston suburb known for its high-end shopping, restaurants, and neighborhoods. Anusara Yoga quickly became one of the most popular yoga systems in the world. In a 2010 interview with a *New York Times* journalist, Friend made the following statement about how Anusara Yoga compares to other yoga systems: "[People know about physically oriented yoga] but as we grow they are going to learn about Anusara. Then people can choose—either they are going to go to a fast-food joint or a fine restaurant" (Swartz 2010). For Friend, yoga, like food, is a consumable product, and his brand, Anusara, signifies better product quality.

Twenty-two years after his 1989 visit to India, Friend was invited to lead the grand finale of the 2011 Wanderlust festival.[2] Bringing Wanderlust to a close, Friend suggested that year's festival was particularly "auspicious" because it fell on the fiftieth anniversary of the death of Nityananda (d. 1961) (Buckner 2011), identified in Siddha Yoga as a former guru of the tradition. In this way, Friend publicly tied his mass-marketed postural yoga brand not just to tantra, but to Siddha Yoga in particular.[3]

All of this raises questions regarding the ways that postural yoga is effectively mass-marketed to large audiences of consumers today. How, after all, did an Ohio-born former financial analyst who grew up in the Houston suburbs become the founder of the most widely consumed tantra-inspired postural yoga system in the world?

In this chapter, I ask and attempt to answer that question by contextualizing Friend and Anusara Yoga within the social milieu of contemporary consumer culture. It turns out that the model of brand image management—branding is systematic and pervasive in contemporary consumer culture—is effective for understanding the popularization of yoga today.[4] Throughout yoga's history, proponents have established and acknowledged authority primarily, though not exclusively, through lineages based on transmission from guru to disciple. However, beginning in the late twentieth century, yoga proponents also established and acknowledged authority by branding yoga.

After a general discussion on branding in consumer culture, I evaluate the context in which three specific systems of yoga became subject to a sequential branding process: selection, introduction, elaboration, and fortification.[5] I suggest that Iyengar Yoga, Siddha Yoga, and Anusara Yoga illustrate how the model of brand image management is effective for understanding a broader phenomenon: the contemporary global popularization of yoga. I trace the steps through which two first-generation yoga entrepreneurs, Iyengar and Muktananda, constructed yoga brands, Iyengar Yoga and Siddha Yoga respectively. I then suggest that Friend is a second-generation yoga entrepreneur who selected from Iyengar Yoga and Siddha Yoga and subsequently introduced, elaborated, and fortified the Anusara Yoga brand. He associated his postural yoga brand with his own persona, modern tantric ideas, and modern biomechanical wares, all of which were attractive to large target audiences of late-twentieth- and early-twenty-first-century consumers. Finally, I suggest that Anusara Yoga is particularly illustrative of contemporary yoga branding not only because of its success as a result of brand image management, but also because of how it illustrates gaffes in yoga brand image management.

"Packaging" Yoga

Numerous twentieth-century events and individuals were significant portents of yoga branding. As noted in Chapter Three, in many areas of the industrialized world, most notably for the current study urban centers in India, North America, and Western Europe, consumers witnessed dramatic increases in access to information about worldviews and practices as well as decreases in the stigma around choosing from a plurality of worldviews and practices to construct individual lifestyles. All of this resulted in a competitive marketplace in which what are often termed *New Age* products were increasingly popular.

Hugh B. Urban suggests that the New Age movement represents an adaptation to consumer culture insofar as it adopts disparate elements from different worldviews based on the needs and concerns of the individual (Urban 2000: 296). Paul Heelas adds that the New Age is "detraditionalized" and emphasizes "spiritual technologies" drawn from various religious traditions (Heelas 1996: 2, 68; see also Albanese 2007: 508). This is compatible with the unique pluralization of the global market in contemporary consumer culture. Individuals do not simply choose from a limited set of religious systems within a particular cultural point of reference, but from entirely different ideological and religious systems, including the modern scientific one. In an effort to meet individual needs, many postural yoga proponents, like those of New Age bodies of religious practice, market postural yoga as a universal and scientific system that anyone can adopt as part of his or her larger worldview and practice. Yoga entrepreneurs and organizations seek to disseminate yoga to the general populace. To do that, yoga needs to stand out in the marketplace among available products and services by being branded or "packaged" in ways that make it seem valuable, accessible, and unique.

Krishnamacharya and Sivananda's students were the first to associate physical fitness methods and aims with yoga in the popular imagination by constructing yoga brands and mass-marketing them to large audiences. With these developments, the aims of postural yoga in the popular imagination came to include modern conceptions of physical fitness, stress reduction, beauty, and overall well-being (de Michelis 2004; Strauss 2005; Albanese 2007; Newcombe 2007; Singleton 2010).

Krishnamacharya had arguably the most impact on postural yoga's entry into the global marketplace, since it was his students, most notably Iyengar, K. Pattabhi Jois, and T.K.V. Desikachar (b. 1938), who constructed yoga brands and most successfully marketed those brands to the general populace in the second half of the twentieth century in urban centers across the world. Some of Sivananda's students were also influential in this regard, especially Vishnudevananda. Other mid-twentieth-century yoga proponents, as noted in Chapter Three, constructed new soteriological yoga systems and marketed them to the general populace. The 1960s provided ideal timing for the global dissemination of such systems, since it witnessed the British-American counterculture and the lifting of immigration restrictions, especially to the United States, the United Kingdom, and France. In turn, several Indian gurus—including Muktananda of Siddha Yoga, Maharishi Mahesh Yogi of Transcendental Meditation, Bhaktivedanta Prabhupada of the International Society for Krishna Consciousness, Mahaprajna of the Jain Terapanth through his mediators, the samanis, and Iyengar of Iyengar Yoga—exploited these robust trends by branding tantric, meditational, devotional, and postural yoga systems and marketing them to large audiences.

Socioeconomic shifts were also significant. The twentieth century featured a shift toward mass production and mass consumption in urban areas across the world, and new groups of consumers increasingly exercised choice with regard to the products and services they purchased (Bocock 1993: 22). In the second half of the twentieth century, economies increasingly shifted from an industrial one based on mass production to a personalized one based on "customized products for individualistic consumers" (Russell 1993: 56). In short, consumer culture came to be based

on individualized products and services. Mike Featherstone descr
this consumer culture:

> In contrast to the designation of the 1950s as an era of grey con-
> formism, a time of *mass* consumption, changes in production
> techniques, market segmentation and consumer demand for a
> wider range of products, are often regarded as making possible
> greater choice (the management of which itself becomes an art
> form)... (Featherstone 2007: 81)

As consumption increasingly pivoted around individual preference, even
religion often became subject to individual choice. Through mass-marketed
books and other media, religious products and services were often not even
tied to particular times and places, such as church on Sunday morning, but
could be practiced anywhere at any time (Einstein 2008: 7).

Today, whether or not certain yoga products and services are consumed
depends in part on whether or not they are linked to consumer desires.
According to Jean Baudrillard, consumers construct the self-identity
they desire by consuming what they think signifies that self-identity
(Baudrillard 2002). This occurs through the use of signs and symbols
(Bocock 1993: 3). Market researchers and advertising campaign managers link products and services to consumer desires by establishing
brand images for everything from dish soaps to sporting goods (Bocock
1993: 22). In other words, branding discourses operate to link consumer
desires to a certain brand's products and services. BULLSHIT

The second half of the twentieth century witnessed an explosion
of sundry yoga brands into the marketplace. Entrepreneurs began to
brand yoga in the same ways other products and services are branded,
by "giving it a name, term, design, symbol, or any other feature that
identifies one seller's good or services as distinct from those of other
sellers" (American Marketing Association 2012). Branding requires
marketers to uniquely package their products by "mythologizing" them,
a process that serves to "position" them in consumers' minds (Einstein
2008: 12). As yoga generates somatic, semantic, and symbolic fields of
meaning meant to appeal to consumer desires, brands seek to signify
those meanings to millions of individuals interested in doing yoga. In
this way, branding mythologizes yoga products and services, ranging
from mats and pants to styles and teachers. And one of the most common themes is that yoga signifies self-development. In other words, it

is a tool that will enable consumers to become better people through physical and psychological transformations (de Michelis 2004; Strauss 2005; Albanese 2007; Newcombe 2007; Singleton 2010).

More than those of any other form of modern yoga, postural yoga brands are widely consumed today. As noted in Chapter Three, this was in part due to the universalization and accessibility of postural yoga. Also, dominant ways of conceptualizing the body in contemporary consumer culture are important for understanding why postural yoga underwent popularization. Elizabeth de Michelis, for example, suggests that, by the mid-twentieth century, postural yoga had conceded to drastic changes in popular mores, which in turn brought about changes in popular ideals of body image and identity (de Michelis 2004: 249; de Michelis cites journalist Horwell 1998: 12). Consumers allocated increasing importance to physical grooming, fitness, and the cultivation of a youthful body (de Michelis 2004: 249). In consumer culture, the inner and outer bodies are "conjoined," meaning that body enhancement is taken to reflect self-development (Featherstone 1991: 171). Consequently, the market for physical culture regimens, in which body enhancement requires rigorous self-control through diet and exercise (Albanese 2007; Singleton 2010), has witnessed robust growth. Furthermore, a biomedical dialect dominates the way people think and talk about their bodies (Turner, Bryan S. 1997: 35). Successful postural yoga entrepreneurs exploit such pop culture trends by managing their brand images in ways that make them represent these ways of conceptualizing the body and self-development. By appropriating popular ideals and trends, postural yoga entrepreneurs have successfully established yoga in the "sports and fitness" market (de Michelis 2004: 249).

Most postural yoga entrepreneurs and organizations prescribe yoga not as an all-encompassing worldview or system of practice, but as one part of self-development that can be consumed in combination with other worldviews and practices. All of this serves to make yoga attractive to large target audiences of consumers who do not want to go to an Indian ashram or seek out a proselytizing guru in order to do yoga. Instead of relying on yoga transmission through the traditional guru–disciple relationship in the isolated context of an ashram, most postural yoga entrepreneurs build large organizations for mass-marketing the easily accessible wares associated with their yoga brands (Fig. 4.1).

Today, most yoga consumers shop for conveniently located postural yoga classes that are open to the general populace and for other yoga

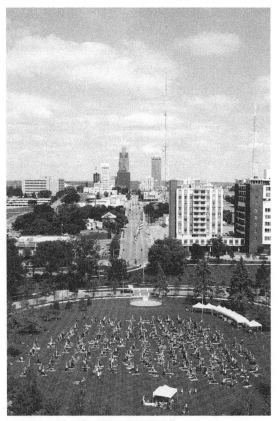

FIGURE 4.1 People practice postural yoga *en masse* during special events around the world each year. For example, practitioners gather annually in twenty cities across the United States to celebrate Yoga Rocks the Park, described as "a locally staffed celebration of community for the whole family promoting peace, giving and wellbeing on a local and global scale" (Yoga Rocks the Park 2014). In this image, hundreds pose together in the *virabhadra asana* (warrior posture) in 2011 at the Yoga Rocks the Park event in Omaha, Nebraska. Photographed by Daniel Muller. (Courtesy of *Esoteric Velvet*, from a story by Meghann Schense, esotericvelvet.com.)

products, such as yoga pants, that are immediately available in local shopping malls or through online retail sites. More generally, consumers have "substantial and unpredictable decision-making power in the selection and use of cultural commodities" (Willis 1990: 137). Entrepreneurs and organizations, in turn, construct brands that they think consumers will buy. Consumers, however, are not the only agents. Rather, the construction of brands is based on a dialectical exchange between the entrepreneurs who produce desires and needs for goods and services and consumers who choose them based on individual preferences (Holt 2002: 71–72). In this way, cultural production is integrated into commodity production and consumption. The result is not a homogenous set of shared meanings and values but rather a heterogeneous culture with various overlapping groups (Arnould and Thompson 2005: 868–869), hence the diversified yoga market today.

The concomitant commodifying processes result in a heterogeneity of ever-new yoga systems. As noted in preceding chapters, change and heterogeneity are not new to the history of yoga, but what differs today is the extent to which the media saturates consumer culture, which brings consumers into near-constant contact with advertising and causes yoga products and services to change and develop at a rate never seen before in its history.

Popularized yoga systems offer similar ends: self-development through physical and psychological transformations (de Michelis 2004; Strauss 2005; Albanese 2007; Newcombe 2007; Singleton 2010). Consequently, the only way for the consumer to differentiate one set of yoga products and services from another is to interpret the idiosyncratic meanings that brands signify. Brands signify different meanings by being packaged differently. The process of differentiating one set of products and services from another is an important process for the consumer, since, as noted above, consumption is entwined with constructing a sense of identity (Giddens 1991; Bocock 1993; Baudrillard 2002). In short, the consumption of yoga products is personal. Consequently, yoga entrepreneurs must manage their brand images in ways that make consumers feel personally connected to them.

In the economic circumstances of market capitalism, however, a personal connection with a product is not usually enough to make it yours. Rather, the consumption of products and services almost always requires the consumer to spend money. The amount of spending on yoga depends largely on brand. A consumer can purchase a pair of yoga pants with an unfamiliar brand at the popular retail store Target for $19.99 or purchase a pair from Lululemon, a high-end yoga-apparel brand that on average charges $98 for yoga pants. On the retail website Amazon, the consumer can choose from a variety of yoga mats with unfamiliar brands for under $20, or she can go to a specialty shop and purchase a stylish Manduka-brand yoga mat, which will cost as much as $100. And all that does not include the cost of yoga classes, which widely range from $5 to over $20 per class. And if a consumer is really dedicated to investing money in yoga, for thousands of dollars she can purchase a spot in a yoga retreat in locations throughout the United States, in Europe, or even in the Bahamas or Brazil, with yoga teachers marketing their own popular brands, such as Bikram Choudhury, whose brand is Bikram Yoga, or Friend and his Anusara Yoga. Spending on yoga is steadily increasing. In the United States alone, spending doubled from $2.95 billion to $5.7 billion from 2004 to 2008 (Macy 2008) and climbed to $10.3 billion between 2008 and 2012 (Macy 2012).

The meaning of yoga is conveyed, however, not only through what products and services yogis choose to purchase but also what they choose *not* to purchase.[6] In other words, consumption can require exchange of money and commodities, and the amount of money spent on commodities largely depends on the brand choices of individual consumers. However, consumption can also lack an exchange of money and commodities. Many contemporary yogis, in fact, oppose the commodification of yoga by consuming free yoga services and rejecting certain yoga products.

For example, the yoga practitioner can now opt out of purchasing a yoga mat altogether or attend donation-based yoga classes. Although I will discuss such phenomena in more detail in Chapter Five, for now it is sufficient to note that they are becoming especially prevalent in New York City, where organizations—most popular of which is the hot yoga brand, Yoga to the People (Yoga to the People 2011a)—that provide donation-based yoga classes or yoga classes that do not require a mat, are growing. Some yogis choose brands of yoga that do not require a mat, such as Laughing Lotus (Laughing Lotus 2012), which has studios in New York and San Francisco, because those brands are believed to better signify the meaning of yoga.

To illustrate how yoga brands signify various meanings, I suggest the reader consider the following example of how this occurs in another area of consumption, that of breakfast. Within a single household a variety of breakfast cereals fill the cabinet as a reflection of the various desires and needs of individual members. In the refrigerator, one may find a variety of options with regard to milk and fruit to layer atop the cereal. Each constructs a unique breakfast option by picking each part to construct a whole suited to individual preferences. One constructs one's breakfast based on what choices signify. A consumer who values health may choose the Kashi-brand whole-grain cereal and skim milk. A consumer who values strength and heroism may choose the Kellogg's-brand cereal box featuring Spiderman. And the consumer who values convenience and social status may skip breakfast cereal altogether and instead stop at Starbucks for one of their recognizably branded cups of coffee to carry into work. Consumers construct individual breakfasts suited to their preferences, and their choices, like all choices in consumer culture, mean more than just the stuff—grains, marshmallows, or caffeine—of the breakfast itself.

In the same way, choices in the area of yoga mean more than just the stuff—teachers, spandex, retreats, mats, or studios—of the products and services themselves. In the yoga market, the process of yoga branding and the process of the economic exchange of yoga commodities are distinct, even though they almost always overlap. Yoga brands are saturated with meaning insofar as they signify what consumers desire and deem valuable, and consumers choose brands based on what they consider the most effective and accessible path to get there.

First-Generation Yoga Brands: Iyengar Yoga and Siddha Yoga

Two yoga brands, Iyengar Yoga and Siddha Yoga, are illustrative of how first-generation yoga entrepreneurs constructed a postural yoga brand and a soteriological yoga brand respectively and marketed them in the late-twentieth-century global marketplace.

In response to the robust trends in the global fitness market, Iyengar selected from Krishnamacharya's aerobic yoga as physical culture and elaborated upon those teachings to create Iyengar Yoga as a physical fitness brand. Iyengar prescribed a rigorous and disciplined form of body maintenance, famously referring to the body as a "temple" and arguing, "[The yogi] conquers the body and renders it a fit vehicle for the soul" (Iyengar 1966: 21). The body is preeminent in Iyengar Yoga: "To the yogi his body is the prime instrument of attainment. If his vehicle breaks down, the traveler cannot go far. If the body is broken by ill-health, the aspirant can achieve little" (Iyengar 1966: 24). He prescribed the use of fitness tools, such as belts, bricks, and ropes, meant to help the yogi "conquer" the body. Iyengar Yoga is convincingly linked to biomedical understandings of the body and can be chosen as one part of self-development that is easily incorporated into personalized fitness regimens (de Michelis 2004: 197–198).

As a consequence of many steps toward elaborating and fortifying his yoga brand, Iyengar succeeded in mass-marketing it in the 1960s and 1970s. Arguably the most significant event in the process of elaborating the brand, Iyengar published his *Light on Yoga* (1966), which also served to fortify the Iyengar Yoga brand as it underwent successful mass marketing. Its biomedical dialect was attractive to many. For example, Iyengar suggests:

> Āsanas have been evolved over the centuries so as to exercise every muscle, nerve and gland in the body. They secure a fine physique, which is strong and elastic without being muscle-bound and they keep the body free from disease. They reduce fatigue and soothe the nerves. But their real importance lies in the way they train and discipline the mind. (Iyengar 1966: 40)

Iyengar's biomedical dialect made postural yoga appealing to a wide array of modern urban individuals. The book also made postural yoga particularly attractive because it included step-by-step instructions so that individuals could choose yoga as one part of their self-development regimens and incorporate it into their lifestyles according to their personal needs and desires—students could choose from a variety of postures and other techniques—without having to give up other lifestyle commitments. Students did not even have to go to a formal yoga class, but instead could do yoga in their own homes. In short, Iyengar Yoga was modern and readily accessible.

Another way that *Light on Yoga* served to elaborate the Iyengar Yoga brand is that it established authority by claiming ties to an ancient yoga transmission. Basically, Iyengar affiliated his postural yoga brand with the yoga tradition presented in the text popularly recognized as the "classical" source on yoga, the *Yoga Sutras*, usually attributed to Patanjali, as well as to later hatha yoga developments. For example, the epigraph to *Light on Yoga* is the following "Prayer":

> I bow before the noblest of sages, Patanjali, who brought serenity of mind by his work on yoga, clarity of speech by his work on grammar and purity of body by his work on medicine.

> I salute Adisvara (the Primeval Lord Siva) who taught first the
> science of Hatha Yoga—a science that stands out as a ladder for
> those who wish to scale the heights of Raja Yoga. (Iyengar 1966)

More recently, Iyengar took additional steps toward elaborating the
Iyengar Yoga brand by associating it with an ancient yoga tradition.
Iyengar Yoga responded to recent debates about yoga's identity with what
Joy Laine calls a "retrenchment" phase of development whereby the tradition seeks "to preserve a distinct identity" (Laine 2011). Iyengar Yoga further associated its form of postural yoga with the yoga tradition presented
in the Yoga Sutras by introducing an invocation to Patanjali at the beginning of each yoga class. Iyengar, however, insists that yoga, although a
part of an ancient South Asian yoga transmission, is not specific to any
religious tradition. Consequently, both the epigraph to *Light on Yoga* and
the use of the invocation to Patanjali at the beginning of classes establish authority through appeals to a culturally situated text, while Iyengar
simultaneously claims that Iyengar Yoga is universally accessible.

In the late 1960s and 1970s, additional events served to fortify the
Iyengar Yoga brand. Yoga classes became available at American YMCAs
when Iyengar's students began to teach it. Iyengar Yoga classes were
readily available in major cities such as Chicago and London. Having
hosted several yoga gurus, including Iyengar, for public seminars in
Chicago, Marilyn Englund began teaching her own yoga classes in 1966
at Chicago-area YMCAs (Leviton 1990: 65). By 1971, she had five hundred fifty students per week in twenty-seven classes (Leviton 1990: 65).
Postural yoga classes also became available at the Clapton Adult Education
Institute in London in 1967. Officials argued that "Instructional classes in
Hatha Yoga need not and should not involve treatment of the philosophy
of Yoga. They can be justified only as a form of 'Keep fit' or physical training" (ILEA Further and Higher Education Sub-Committee Papers 1968,
quoted in Newcombe 2007). Iyengar's students' yoga classes at American
YMCAs and London institutions were thoroughly postural and were
deemed beneficial for a variety of consumers regardless of other religious
or lifestyle commitments.

Most significant to the fortification of Iyengar Yoga, in 1975 Iyengar
established the Ramamani Iyengar Memorial Yoga Institute in Pune. The
Institute, which functioned as the center for teacher training, greatly aug-
mented the amount of yoga teachers getting official training in Iyengar
Yoga. It became the headquarters from which to disseminate Iyengar

Yoga (de Michelis 2004: 200), and it "locked in" consumers, meaning it decreased the likelihood that they would pursue some other yoga ware in the marketplace, since they had made an investment of energy, time, and money in Iyengar Yoga.[7] In this way, the Iyengar Yoga brand could be constructed, marketed, and perpetuated across product lines. In short, it could be managed more effectively.

By 1990, a family of senior Iyengar Yoga teachers, the Mehtas, could report: "[Iyengar] has several million students all over the world following his method. There are Iyengar Institutes and centers in the US, the UK, Europe, Australia, Canada, Israel, Japan, New Zealand, and South Africa, as well as India" (Mehta, Mehta, and Mehta 1990: 9). Since then, Iyengar has established the following Iyengar Yoga Institutions: the Light on Yoga Research Trust, which serves to propagate Iyengar Yoga primarily through funding research on it; the Iyengar Yogashraya, a major Iyengar Yoga center in Mumbai, India; and the Youth's Offerings to Guruji, which serves to propagate Iyengar Yoga primarily through publishing books and producing other Iyengar Yoga products, such as belts and bricks (Ramamani Iyengar Memorial Yoga Institute 2009a). Today, there are thousands of Iyengar Yoga teachers and millions of practitioners in over seventy countries across the world (Ramamani Iyengar Yoga Institute 2009b). Basically, Iyengar Yoga has undergone continuous exponential growth.

Muktananda constructed a very different yoga brand than Iyengar Yoga.[8] In 1960s India, Muktananda selected from the teachings of his guru, Nityananda, and philosophical and practical traditions that pre-existed him, especially premodern hatha yoga, Vedanta, and Kashmir Shaivism, in his construction of a unique persona and set of tantric spiritual wares, which he enveloped under the brand name *Siddha Yoga*. Siddha Yoga signified God-realization and was known for its democratic experiential approach to spirituality. *Shaktipat diksha*, that initiatory ritual through which the guru awakened the disciple to God-realization, was available to everyone.

Though Muktananda's understanding of shaktipat was akin to those found in premodern hatha yoga contexts, his method of disseminating it was not. Muktananda introduced Siddha Yoga to disciples at his ashram, Shree Gurudev Ashram, which resembled a European- or American-style retreat center and hosted large numbers of disciples from around the world. Disciples could choose the extent of their commitment, ranging from becoming a permanent monastic member of Muktananda's community, where Siddha Yoga functioned as an all-encompassing worldview and system of practice, to incorporating Siddha Yoga into their diverse spiritual repertoire.

Based on Muktananda's success in attracting disciples, one could judge him to be an astute entrepreneur. Aware that the global market for spiritual wares required marketers to calculate the costs to the brand for wares associated with unpopular ideas or practices, Muktananda elaborated Siddha Yoga by publicly embracing the popular dimensions of tantra, such as *bhakti* or "devotion" and meditation, rather than the esoteric dimensions, such as the ritual use of intoxicants or sex, that required the practitioner to intentionally transgress normative ethical and purity standards in order to become aware of the reality of nonduality.[9] In short, Siddha Yoga was the product of a process of carefully selecting from tantra and Vedanta as well as contemporary dominant ethical standards for marketability.

For example, Muktananda carefully selected from tantric scriptural sources, embracing exoteric dimensions while eschewing esoteric, transgressive ones. Describing Muktananda and his successor, Chidvilasananda's, use of one tantric scripture, the *Kularnava Tantra*, that includes certain transgressive elements, Douglas Renfrew Brooks comments that they "cite frequently *but selectively*" since "ethical preconditions create criteria that inform the Siddha Yoga guru's scriptural choices" (Brooks, Douglas Renfrew 1997: 334).

Muktananda also selected the dominant normative ethical standards of late-twentieth-century urban environments where democratic religious ideals prevailed. Theoretically, Siddha Yoga was a democratic movement. Although the disciple relied on the grace of the guru, all devotees were equally dependent in this way. Furthermore, all devotees had equal access to Siddha Yoga teachings and practices, were required to perform right actions out of self-effort, and were viewed as having God within them.[10] Muktananda thus argued that Siddha Yoga stood out from traditional or "orthodox" yoga systems.[11]

In the 1970s, Muktananda fortified the Siddha Yoga brand with his world tours. Muktananda went out to urban centers in search of disciples, actively marketing the Siddha Yoga brand. In 1974, he introduced the Intensive, a choreographed retreat where initiates received shaktipat *en masse*. This made the bestowal of shaktipat to hundreds—and today thousands—of people at a time efficient, cost-effective, and available for immediate consumption.[12] By commodifying shaktipat in this way, especially with regard to charging for admission to an Intensive, Muktananda "locked in" consumers.

Consumers' commitment to Siddha Yoga, however, cannot be reduced to consumer lock-in. The testimonies of Siddha Yoga practitioners suggest that, more than anything else, long-term commitment to Siddha Yoga was a result of what it provided in terms of a remystification of the world. Spiritual seekers associated the Siddha Yoga brand with Muktananda, the godman perceived as a *siddha* or "perfected master," and with shaktipat, which involved an experience of nothing less than God.

Muktananda took additional steps toward fortifying the Siddha Yoga brand by supporting Siddha Yoga centers, which provided a sense of group identity to individuals who did not have regular direct contact with the guru himself. In 1975, he established the SYDA (Siddha Yoga Dham Associates) Foundation, the organization responsible for the financial and organizational infrastructure of Siddha Yoga outside of India. Organizational developments included the introduction of Siddha Yoga courses and teacher training programs as well as establishing departments for the publication of Siddha Yoga books. All of this enabled the construction, marketing, and perpetuation of the Siddha Yoga brand across product lines.

Successful brand image management resulted in thousands of people from urban areas across the world choosing Siddha Yoga. To its consumers, Siddha Yoga signified a virtuous life, a remystification of the world, and a strong sense of belonging to an organized community. And Muktananda made initiation into the Siddha Yoga life readily accessible in the form of shaktipat, conveniently delivered by means of the Intensive, where up to hundreds of people at a time could have direct contact with the guru himself.

Brand success, however, did decline after accusations of improprieties against Muktananda following his death—Muktananda was accused of having sex with young female disciples, including some teenagers (see Caldwell 2001; Urban 2003: 243–250; Jain 2014b: 203–207). Yet Muktananda's successor, Chidvilasananda, and her disciples have managed to refortify the brand through various strategies to keep it competing in the global market for spiritual wares (on these strategies, see Caldwell 2001; Jain 2014b: 203–207). Although Siddha Yoga and other soteriological yoga brands have not succeeded in attracting large numbers of consumers to the extent that popular postural yoga brands have done so, today there are Siddha Yoga ashrams or centers in thirty countries worldwide (SYDA Foundation 2012), and Friend is only one among thousands of contemporary yoga consumers to choose Siddha Yoga.

A Second-Generation Yoga Brand: Anusara Yoga

On the one hand, Iyengar and Muktananda, first-generation yoga entrepreneurs, selected from the nonbranded yoga systems of Krishnamacharya and Nityananda respectively to construct yoga brands that would be mass-marketed to the general populace. On the other hand, Friend, a second-generation yoga entrepreneur, selected from previously existing yoga brands, Iyengar Yoga and Siddha Yoga, to construct the Anusara Yoga brand. Having selected and introduced his yoga brand in the 1990s, he elaborated and fortified it throughout the early 2000s. Successful brand image management resulted in hundreds of thousands of people from urban areas across the world choosing Anusara Yoga in what was now a diversified global yoga market.

Before introducing his yoga brand, Friend had a laudable yoga career. He studied with one of the most famous living postural yoga teachers, Iyengar, and spent four years on the Board of Directors of the Iyengar Yoga National Association. In 1995, he returned to the Ramamani Iyengar Memorial Yoga Institute for another one-month intensive yoga program. He also studied with other world-famous teachers, including Desikachar, Patabhi Jois, and Indra Devi. None of them affected him as powerfully as Chidvilasananda, the guru of Siddha Yoga (Williamson 2014: 215). Friend maintained ties to Siddha Yoga—he spent almost every summer from 1992 to 2004 living and teaching in the Hatha Yoga Department at the Siddha Yoga Shree Muktananda Ashram in South Fallsburg, New York (Friend 2009b).[13]

All of Friend's hours of study under various yoga masters significantly influenced his selection process as he constructed his own idiosyncratic yoga system. More than anything else, Friend embraced the rigorous physical fitness and biomechanical dimensions of Iyengar Yoga and the nondual tantric philosophy of Siddha Yoga. After realizing the conflict between Siddha Yoga philosophy and Iyengar Yoga, which maintained the dualist philosophy of the Yoga Sutras—Iyengar suggests, for instance, "The yogi knows that he is different from his body, which is a temporary house for his spirit" (Iyengar 1995: 33)—and emphasized physical fitness at what Friend perceived to be the loss of spirituality (Williamson 2014: 217), Friend set out to construct his own form of tantra-inspired postural yoga, which he thought would resolve the perceived incompatibilities between Siddha Yoga and Iyengar Yoga.

When Friend introduced Anusara Yoga in 1997, the brand represented a mix of postural yoga, a tantric nondual philosophy, and a life-affirming and lighthearted approach that is premised on the idea "that everything in this world is an embodiment of Supreme Consciousness, which at its essence pulsates with goodness and the highest bliss" (Anusara, Inc. 2009a). Based on his years studying Iyengar Yoga, Friend adopted certain biomechanical principles but, based on his years studying Siddha Yoga, gave them a nondualist tantric spin, arguing that their aim was "to bring the body into alignment with the Optimal Blueprint" (Friend 2009a: 39). In addition to the Anusara philosophy, the variety of books available through Anusara Yoga's website, which features books on tantric philosophy as well as books on biomedical perspectives on anatomy, physiology, and fitness (Anusara, Inc. 2009b), evidences Friend's selection from both Iyengar's postural yoga and Siddha Yoga's soteriological yoga.

All of Friend's selective and elaborative strategies resulted in one of the most successful yoga brands in the world. Friend convinced hundreds of thousands of consumers to choose his yoga brand over others, and the demand for his products quickly went global. What made Friend's yoga brand stand out most was that it signified the idea that goodness is present in everyone in a life-affirming way. According to Friend, "After studying everything, tantra is not only the most elegant and sophisticated system, but it's the one that aligns with my heart because it sees that the very essence of life is joy or love and that there's a goodness to life" (Williamson 2014: 216). According to Lola Williamson, who conducted several interviews with Friend and his students, "Positively affirming his students with lightness and humor quickly became the hallmark of Friend's teaching style" (Williamson 2014: 217).

In 1998, Friend took an important step toward fortifying his brand when he developed instructions for how to teach Anusara Yoga and published them as the *Anusara Teacher Training Manual* (2009). With over a thousand licensed teachers worldwide, Anusara became one of the most widely consumed yoga systems in the transnational yoga market.

In addition to consumers who attended yoga studios where teachers taught Anusara Yoga, hundreds and sometimes thousands of people at a time gathered at yoga workshops, conferences, and festivals to hear Friend dispense his teachings on yoga as fitness and spirituality. Friend offered workshops all over the United States and the world at destinations as widespread as Taipei, Tokyo, Copenhagen, and Munich.

Friend's steps toward fortifying the Anusara Yoga brand locked in consumers. Committed students spent thousands of dollars on yoga classes, teacher training workshops, and traveling costs, not to mention other Anusara Yoga products, ranging from the Anusara yoga clothing line to Anusara Yoga mats and water bottles (Anusara Inc. 2009d). Friend even collaborated with the fitness clothing giant Adidas and the yoga accessories giant Manduka.

Consumers' commitment to Anusara Yoga, however, cannot be reduced to the phenomenon of consumer lock-in; Anusara Yoga, in short, was more than just its commodities. Based on numerous interviews with Anusara Yoga practitioners, Williamson suggests that Anusara Yoga provided a strong sense of community and meaning for individuals who rejected traditional institutionalized religious contexts (2014: 218–225). Friend offered a yoga system that was accessible to a large audience, since its life-affirming, lighthearted approach, like most successful consumer goods, was not all-encompassing and instead could be integrated as one part of a larger worldview or lifestyle. Furthermore, Friend appealed to those consumers who desired a form of yoga that involved positive affirmation while simultaneously avoiding doing so at the loss of an emphasis on physical fitness.

Anusara Yoga was also successful because, in a way similar to Muktananda, Friend elaborated the Anusara Yoga brand by publicly embracing the exoteric dimensions of "classical" yoga and tantra, such as postures, breathing exercises, and ethical guidelines, rather than the esoteric dimensions that required the practitioner to renounce or deliberately transgress normative standards. Unlike the Siddha Yoga gurus, Friend emphasized physical fitness instead of unyielding guru devotion and mystical experience, but in accordance with the Siddha Yoga gurus, Friend never publicly prescribed transgressive techniques. Rather, he prescribed the strict ethical guidelines as articulated for all Anusara Yoga consumers on the Anusara website (Anusara, Inc. 2009c). For example, the guidelines include Friend's modern interpretation of "classical" yoga ethics, such as the following:

Ahimsa (Non-harming): Loving kindness to others, not blocking or obstructing the flow of Nature, compassion, mercy, gentleness, commonly translated as non-violence.

Satya (Truthfulness): Being genuine and authentic to our inner nature, having integrity, honesty, being honorable, not lying, not concealing the truth, not downplaying or exaggerating (Anusara, Inc. 2009c).

They also include "other" yoga ethical guidelines, including:

Be welcoming to all students regardless of gender, race, religion, creed, nationality, cultural background, or sexual preference.

Give feedback by first looking for what is right—the beauty, the light, and the positive in people and things—instead of the ugliness, the darkness, or what is wrong. In this way you will always give the student the benefit of the doubt.

By 2012, because it had successfully signified the meaning of yoga for many consumers, Anusara Yoga was producing millions of dollars a year in revenue, which facilitated exponential growth. That year, Friend was in the middle of one of his world tours, which were important for fortifying his yoga brand. This tour was titled *Igniting the Center* and began in Encinitas, California, a yoga epicenter, in honor of the new headquarters for Anusara Yoga, simply called "The Center," that Friend was building there. But as Friend enjoyed a spotlight in the postural yoga world for his success as the founder of a growing yoga organization and for what was perceived as his virtuous character, he and his yoga brand became marred in scandals. He was accused of transgressing the ethical guidelines that Anusara Yoga prescribed when he made what were perceived as unethical personal and financial decisions.

The accusations can be summarized as follows: Friend led a Wiccan coven and had sex with female members; Friend had numerous sexual relationships with married Anusara employees and teachers; Friend violated federal regulations regarding employee benefits by suddenly freezing Anusara, Inc.'s pension fund; and finally, Friend put his employees at legal risk by arranging for them to accept packages of marijuana meant for his personal use (Yoga Dork 2012b).[14]

Suspicion that the accusations were true grew as people learned that four of Anusara Yoga's most senior teachers—Christina Sell, Darren Rhodes, Elena Brower, and Amy Ippoliti—had recently resigned one by one, citing "professional differences" (Yoga Dork 2012b). Soon after the accusations went public, more of Anusara's most loyal consumers abandoned Anusara Yoga. Two additional senior teachers, Noah Maze and Bernadette Birney, resigned, and Maze stepped down from his position on an interim committee that Friend established to ensure Anusara's survival from the onslaught of the scandals (Yoga Dork 2012b). On her website, Birney added to the scandals, claiming that Friend "decided to 'heal' his students with 'sex therapy'" (Birney 2012).

With the threat of Friend's alleged gaffes permanently damaging the Anusara Yoga brand image, Friend confirmed that he had had sexual relationships with married employees and teachers and that Anusara, Inc. had violated federal regulations regarding employee pension funds (Lewis 2012). Friend also wrote the following to Anusara Yoga teachers:

> The central issue now is that the wonderful image and reputation of Anusara yoga has been severely stained in the minds of some, since my personal behavior has been perceived to be out of integrity with Anusara ethics...the disharmony between my personal image and the values of our school needs to be reconciled, if Anusara is to properly heal...we are exploring scenarios in which the company is restructured to give teachers more voice and representation not only in areas of brand, ethics and curriculum, but also in the governance and direction of the company itself. (Yoga Dork 2012a)

He added, "We must all remember that any missteps by me do not invalidate any of the greatness of the Anusara yoga method" (Yoga Dork 2012a).

Like Muktananda's successor, Chidvilasananda, and her disciples, Friend had to refortify his declining brand image that resulted from the founder's transgressions. To do that, Friend announced the appointment of Michal Lichtman as CEO of the new "teacher-run, nonprofit organization—the Anusara Yoga School," adding that Friend himself would remain only "founder, student, and teacher of Anusara yoga" (Yoga Dork 2012c).

Some journalistic accounts of the scandals assumed that such changes would make a difference to Anusara Yoga's success in the global market. Stewart J. Lawrence suggested in *The Huffington Post* that the Anusara Yoga situation reflected the reality for the entire yoga industry, whose future is grim due to the dominance of "charismatic, guru-based governing structures" rather than "more modern and democratic" ones (Lawrence 2012). This suspicion that the guru model is an extreme form of authoritarianism that inevitably leads to demise is not new. In 1993, for example, Joel Kramer and Diana Alstad warned against the dangers of the guru–disciple relationship, suggesting that it displays "the seductions, predictable patterns, and corruptions contained in any essentially authoritarian form" and "the epitome of surrender to a living person, and thus clearly exhibits what it means to trust another more than oneself" (Kramer and Alstad xiii).

I would suggest, however, that surrender to a guru and his or her spiritual wares is not necessarily quantitatively or qualitatively different than surrender to a brand, in part for its associations with a particular person, whether a self-proclaimed "guru," CEO, or simply a celebrity. Friend was not, after all, the Anusara Yoga guru. Even though Friend used the term *kula* (Sanskrit for "family") to refer to the Anusara Yoga community— a term traditionally applied to disciples gathered around a guru—he rejected the label, preferring instead to call himself the *founder* and (until the 2012 restructuring) *general manager* of Anusara. But that does not mean the infallible attributes often associated with the term *guru* have not been attributed to him. Until the scandals of 2012, Friend had been considered the paragon of virtue within the Anusara community.

But even if Friend *functioned* in certain ways as a guru for the Anusara community, his relationship to the Anusara brand is not different than the relationship of other popular persons to particular brands. Although, as an entrepreneur, Friend constructed a brand and marketed it successfully, he may have also destroyed it. At the very least, he damaged the Anusara Yoga brand image, which illustrates a key dimension of yoga brand image management: The type of yoga one does and what it signifies are not the only things that determine steps toward consumer lock-in. What one's teacher or the founder of one's yoga brand of choice signifies also matters. In other words, yoga brands often signify persons as well as styles or values. In this way, yoga entrepreneurs' relationship to their brands is similar to the relationship of other popular persons to particular brands—think Steve Jobs and the Apple brand. In the same way that Jobs was believed to have abilities beyond mundane marketing skills, Friend was considered to have special insight into the nature of yoga and its path to self-development. When brands signify persons in these ways, it helps the brand images.

Friend's associations with Anusara Yoga were not helping the brand image, and eventually Friend abandoned Anusara Yoga altogether in favor of a new yoga brand: Sridaiva Yoga. Friend left Houston and fled to Denver, Colorado, where he has been elaborating the Sridaiva Yoga brand, which he markets as "an accessible postural system for everyone" (Friend 2012). It is yet to be known whether the steps toward disassociating the Anusara Yoga brand from the person of John Friend or Friend's efforts to market the new Sridaiva Yoga will successfully draw more consumers to either yoga brand.

Conclusion

In the late twentieth century, as economies in urban areas across the world increasingly shifted toward the production and consumption of customized products based on individual consumers' desires and needs, yoga became subject to branding processes. Yoga brands signified the dominant physical and psychological self-developmental desires and needs of many contemporary consumers.

Two first-generation yoga entrepreneurs, Iyengar and Muktananda, constructed early yoga brands, Iyengar Yoga and Siddha Yoga respectively. Iyengar selected from the unbranded yoga system of Krishnamacharya and mass-marketed a postural yoga brand that represented physical fitness, modern biomechanics, and well-being. Muktananda selected from the unbranded yoga system of his guru, Nityananda, Vedanta, and Kashmir Shaivism, and mass-marketed a soteriological yoga brand that provided a remystification of the world and what was perceived as a virtuous guru figure.

Friend, a second-generation yoga entrepreneur, selected from Iyengar Yoga and Siddha Yoga and subsequently introduced, elaborated, and fortified the Anusara Yoga brand. By successfully constructing a brand that signified health, the affirmation of life, lightheartedness, and community, he succeeded in the competitive global yoga market, although numerous gaffes in brand image management, involving what were perceived as Friend's transgressions of Anusara Yoga ethical guidelines, damaged the Anusara Yoga brand image.

The cases of Iyengar Yoga, Siddha Yoga, and Anusara Yoga illustrate how yoga brands are saturated with meaning insofar as they signify what consumers deem valuable. That often includes certain persons deemed to be paragons of virtue or style. They also illustrate that consumers choose based on what they consider the most effective and accessible path—or brand—to get there.

5

Postural Yoga as a Body of Religious Practice

As Durkheim pointed out, anything can become sacred,
so why not the "profane" goods of capitalism?
—MIKE FEATHERSTONE (2007: 119)

— Wuhh7?

TODAY POSTURAL YOGA is a part of pop culture, and brand-name yoga studios, mats, and clothing are easily accessible in many urban locations around the world, where yoga is almost *de rigueur*. A modern question that arises in response to the widespread accessibility of yoga products and services is whether or not they should be subject to state regulation, and determining what qualifies is tricky, especially when religious freedom could be perceived as impeded upon. But is postural yoga *religious*?

Consider regulatory attempts in Texas.[1] Until the end of the first decade of the twenty-first century, Texas approached the regulation of yoga as it approached the regulation of religious institutions and organizations: It refrained. But in early 2010, the Texas Workforce Commission (TWC) informed the program directors of yoga teacher training programs across Texas that they might be running career schools as defined by Chapter 132 of the Texas Education Code.[2] Arguing that the regulation of career schools benefits consumers by monitoring programs, ensuring that they are legitimate businesses, and providing an avenue for student complaints, the TWC requested directors to choose one of the following: Apply and secure a career school license at the cost of up to $3,000 per year, close teacher training programs altogether, file for an exemption and secure it, or face a $50,000 fine. They gave directors fourteen days to comply.

To be clear, there was no law, nor was the TWC attempting to establish a law, regulating yoga teacher training curriculum. In other words, the TWC did not challenge nor did it provide guidelines for curriculum. Yoga Alliance, a North American education and support organization, did and continues to set forth the normative teacher training curriculum guidelines for the Texas yoga community and the American and Canadian ones at large (see Yoga Alliance 2013).[3] Yoga Alliance keeps a Yoga Teachers' Registry and a Registry of Yoga Schools in which it maintains an inventory of those individuals trained and those programs training according to the organization's minimum standards and curriculum. But even those standards and curriculum are not uniformly adopted in teacher training programs across Texas, and yoga teacher training would continue to vary whether or not the state required career school licensing. Furthermore, programs that directors identified as religious or avocational as well as programs that did not offer marketing or business classes, lasted less than twenty-four hours, did not result in a degree or certificate, and cost less than $500 would have been exempt from the licensing requirement.

Nevertheless, concerned that the TWC's requirement would have had undesirable effects on the Texas yoga community, many yogis mobilized against it. Beginning in 2009, Jennifer Buergermeister, a local yoga practitioner, teacher, studio owner, and advocate, led a Texas movement opposing laws that require teacher training programs to be licensed by the state. Participants in the movement argued that this would be the first step toward requiring all yoga teachers to obtain state licenses. Most importantly, they argued that smaller, locally owned studios and programs would not be able to survive under the restrictions and costs proposed by the TWC, which they suggested would result in higher costs for teacher training and classes, less diversity in the community, and the "corporatization" of yoga.

Opponents added that the regulation of yoga teacher training would make no difference with regard to public safety or public good; argued that states sought to regulate yoga for the sake of revenue alone—it is entirely plausible that yoga, which according to a 2012 study (Macy 2012) has become an over $10 billion industry, was targeted for its potential as a source of revenue; and pointed to the fact that, like yoga, practices deemed avocational or recreational, such as martial arts, sewing, and physical fitness, were exempt from state regulation. Yogis added that, by targeting yoga and imposing a requirement that would affect small businesses more than corporate ones, licensing requirements would limit free enterprise, which is acceptable only when the public good or safety is at stake.

Opponents of state regulation in Texas hired an attorney and a lobby-ist to work on their behalf. Conversations culminated in the formation of a coalition, the Texas Yoga Association (TYA), to advocate against state regulation of yoga.[4] They also wrote letters, made calls to their legislators, and collected over a thousand signatures for a petition.

Efforts to stop the regulation of yoga resulted in the introduction of two bills in the Texas legislature. In May 2011, Texas Governor Rick Perry signed SB 1176 (see State of Texas 2011c) into law. The bill excluded yoga from the definition of "post-secondary education," thus exempting yoga teacher training programs from career school licensing requirements. The second bill, HB 1839 (see State of Texas 2011b), also signed into law in 2011, amended the definition of "career school" to exclude anyone who provides recreational classes that do not lead to an educational credential.

The Texas yogis were not the only Americans who opposed regula-tion of yoga. Yogis vocally opposed attempts to impose sales taxes on yoga classes in Connecticut, Washington, and Missouri. In Virginia, protesters against the state regulation of yoga studios filed a suit alleging that regu-lation would violate First Amendment rights to free exercise of religion. Sometimes opponents of state regulation of yoga were successful. After the New York State Education Department tried to assess fines on and to require permits from yoga teacher training programs, for example, a group of yogis mobilized and responded with legislation that exempted yoga teacher training programs from the licensing requirement.

When one looks closely at the opposition to the regulation of yoga, one finds that it is infused with religious discourse. In fact, religious under-standings of yoga have everything to do with the politics of yoga and the reasons why, for many serious practitioners of yoga, nobody is entitled to regulate it.

Postural yogis frequently avoid categorizing yoga as *religion*.[5] Many postural yogis prefer to categorize it as *spiritual* or invoke other nonexplic-itly religious terms to describe it. Following Perry's signing of SB 1176, for example, Buergermeister exclaimed, "This is a huge victory for the Yoga community in Texas. Regulating Yoga as a career school detracted from its rightful place as a spiritual and philosophical tradition" (Texas Yoga Association 2009). J. Brown, a postural yoga advocate in New York, opposed state regulation of yoga because yoga is "sacred," is an "all-encompassing whole Truth," and functions to explore the "self, health, and life" (Brown,

J. 2005).[6] Yoga studio owner, and instructor Bruce Roger, an opponent of the taxation of yoga classes in Missouri, definitively stated, "Yoga is a spiritual practice. It's not a purchase" (Huffstutter 2009).

Many postural yogis avoid the category *religion* because it connotes an authoritative institution or doctrine in the popular imagination. T. K. V. Desikachar suggests, "Yoga is not a religion and should not [affiliate] with any religion" because yoga does not have a doctrine concerning the existence of God (Catalfo n.d.). *Yoga Journal* journalist Phil Catalfo suggests that yoga is best categorized as spirituality, not religion, because religion is "the organizational structure we give to our individual and collective spiritual processes: the rituals, doctrines, prayers, chants, and ceremonies, and the congregations that come together to share them," and yoga has no "religious obligations" with regard to such things (Catalfo n.d.).

Many postural yogis share a vision of religion that narrowly defines it primarily in terms of shared belief. That vision has been privileged among Protestants and Catholics since the seventeenth century (Smith, Wilfred Cantwell, 1991 [1962]). The implication is that a person cannot rationally adopt two or more religions at the same time because that would entail commitment to different, and incompatible, belief systems.

As a scholar of religion, however, I think more broadly about what counts as religious than most people do.[7] That broader assessment results in a vision of postural yoga as a body of practice that is profoundly religious. I use *body of religious practice* here to refer to a set of behaviors characterized by the following: They are treated as sacred, set apart from the ordinary or mundane;[8] they are grounded in a shared ontology or worldview (although that ontology may or may not provide a metanarrative or all-encompassing worldview); they are grounded in a shared axiology or set of values or goals concerned with resolving weakness, suffering, or death; and the above qualities are reinforced through narrative and ritual.

I begin by covering and eventually rejecting some outside observers' profoundly trivializing reactions to postural yoga that do not take it seriously as a body of religious practice but rather reduce it to a mere commodity of global market capitalism or to no more than impotent borrowings from or "rebrandings" of traditional religious products. Such observers provide accounts of postural yoga that do not take insider perspectives on postural yoga seriously. I respond to three problems with these trivializing reactions by providing and analyzing exempla from postural yoga in a way that takes insider perspectives seriously. All of this amounts to a fuller, more adequate account of postural yoga, an account that conveys its many religious qualities.

Postural Yoga as a Mere Commodity of Global Market Capitalism

One response to postural yoga has been to ignore emic accounts (accounts from the perspectives of those who live *inside* the relevant body of practice, accepting its basic worldview, rituals, and values) and to instead analyze postural yoga based exclusively on etic accounts (accounts from where people live *outside* the relevant body of practice).[9]

Unsurprisingly, when it comes to scholarly analyses of yoga products and services, especially those that self-identify as "tantric," some thinkers immediately write off emic accounts as unworthy of serious consideration. Well-known scholar of yoga and tantra David Gordon White, for example, makes the following assessment of modern tantra:

> Then there are the Western dilettantes, the self-proclaimed Tantric entrepreneurs, who have hitched their elephant-wagons to the New Age star to peddle a dubious product called Tantric Sex, which they (and their clientele) assume to be all there ever was to Tantra. (White 2000: 4)

He further describes these capitalist "dilettantes" as "the for-profit purveyors of Tantric Sex, who have no compunctions about appropriating a misguided nineteenth-century polemic to peddle their shoddy wares" (White 2000: 5).

Likewise, some exclusively etic accounts of postural yoga amount to broadly targeted refusals to take it seriously as a body of religious practice, since, from their perspectives, it can be reduced to impotent borrowings from ancient yoga traditions put in service to capitalist values. According to such thinkers, postural yoga represents a mere commodification that exploits or distracts from what is perceived as the ancient, traditional, and homogonous yoga tradition.

Accomplished yoga scholar Georg Feuerstein, for example, refused to seriously analyze postural yoga as a body of religious practice. He considered "the popularization of yoga as potentially destructive of the yogic heritage" since it embodies "distortions" of yoga (Feuerstein

2003). He added that postural yoga is inauthentic because "fitness and health," some of its aims, "are simply not final objectives of traditional yoga," and suggested that those interested in yoga should focus on "The 'lost' teachings of yoga—that is, the authentic teachings as found in the traditional literature and as imbued with life by living masters" (Feuerstein 2003).

The study *Selling Spirituality* (2005) by Jeremy Carrette and Richard King serves as perhaps the paragon of the tendency to write off postural yoga as nothing more than mere commodification. The authors target the "big business" of "spirituality," including postural yoga. Though the authors claim that their concern is with the sociopolitical consequences of the "spiritual marketplace" and not with the truth, authenticity, or the question of "what counts as real spirituality," their analysis of the "spiritual marketplace" is framed as the capitalist "takeover," "commercialization," and "replacement" of religion (2005). This opposition between capitalist commodification and religion amounts to an assessment of what counts as real religion. Carrette and King's reduction of pop culture spiritual products to the mere commodification of what were traditional religious wares—"What is being sold to us as radical, trendy and transformative spirituality in fact produces little in the way of a significant change in one's lifestyle or fundamental behaviour patterns" (2005: 5)—frames spirituality as distinct from religion and presumes, therefore, that practices identified by insiders as *spiritual* cannot function as a legitimate body of religious practice.

Carrette and King warn:

> [T]he ideologies of consumerism and business enterprise are now infiltrating more and more aspects of our lives. The result of this shift has been an erasure of the wider social and ethical concerns associated with religious traditions and communities and the subordination of "the religious" and the ethical to the realm of economics. (2005: 4–5)

In short, there is no religious substance to self-proclaimed spiritualities; rather, they exclusively serve to reinforce capitalist values.

On the term *spirituality*, Carrette and King add, "The very ambiguity of the term means that it can operate across different social and interest groups and in capitalist terms, function to establish a market niche". (2005: 31). Spiritualities, according to this vision, redefine religious categories, which amounts to "rebranding" ancient traditions (2005: 16). This is especially the case with spiritual brands that marketers claim represent Asian spiritualities, such as postural yoga. In reality, Carrette and King suggest, they represent nothing more than the "very western cultural *obsession* with the individual self and a distinct lack of interest in compassion, the disciplining of desire, self-less service to others and questions of social justice" (2005: 114).

Carrette and King point to postural yoga as an especially apt example, since it radically differs from its claimed origins, the ancient South Asian systems of Patanjala Yoga and hatha yoga. The authors suggest that postural yoga separates yoga from its religio-philosophical, ascetic, and ethical dimensions (2005: 117–118), and, quoting Kimberley Lau, suggest that postural yoga relies on physical practice exclusively and at the loss of a "complete" lifestyle (2005: 117; see Lau 2000: 104). The authors add that postural yoga ignores the selfless ethical agenda in service to society and the environment that they believe characterizes ancient yoga traditions:

> What [Hindu yoga and Buddhist "inner technologies of the self"] share in common is a comprehensive and radical critique of the conventional ego-driven and particularized self that sees itself as the all-important focus of our lives—as the centre of our universes. This challenge to our everyday understanding of the self and its desires is lost however when yoga is transformed in modern western societies into an individualized spirituality of the self, or, as we are increasingly seeing, repackaged as a cultural commodity to be sold to the "spiritual consumer." (116)

Carrette and King continue to elaborate upon these homogenizing and essentializing visions of both ancient and contemporary postural yoga:

> [I]t is clear that the metaphysical, institutional and societal dimensions of ancient yoga traditions are largely lost in the translation and popularization of yoga in the West…An arduous path to enlightenment and liberation from the cycle of rebirths through the conquest of selfish desires becomes yet another modern method for pacifying and accommodating individuals to the world in which they find themselves (2005: 119–120).

They add:

> Whatever their fundamental worldview, all forms of Hindu yoga
> reject the motivational structure upon which consumerism is pred-
> icated—namely identification with the embodied individual self
> and acting to further its own self-interest. (2005: 121)

In other words, premodern yoga "involves a reorientation *away* from the
concerns of the individual and towards an appreciation of the wider social
and cosmic dimensions of our existence" (2005: 121). This, according to
Carrette and King, is the opposite of what characterizes contemporary
postural yoga, which is construed as nothing more than a capitalist enterprise. Carrette and King lament, "Yoga essentially became a form of
exercise and stress-relief to be classified alongside the other health and
'sports-related' practices and fads of the late twentieth century" (2005: 119).

Insider Visions of Postural Yoga

Carrette and King (2005) contribute to a growing literature that evaluates
the contemporary buying and selling of spiritual products (see, e.g., Roof
1999 and Lau 2000). They are concerned exclusively with who profits in
the market and the ethical problems of the capitalist marketplace and provide important insights into the ways that spiritual products reflect adaptations and responses to trends in the global capitalist market. Yet, along
with others who dismiss popular spiritualities as mere commodities of
market capitalism, they simultaneously fail to account for the religious
functions and meanings of those products. Consequently, their visions
of pop culture spiritualities, including those of postural yoga, are largely
incongruent with and fail to account for the visions of insiders.

Trivializing approaches to postural yoga, such as the one Carrette and
King offer, betray the following three assumptions about what should
be taken seriously as bodies of religious practice: What counts as sacred
should be opposed to the profane or mundane, should be the good (in
a modern ethical sense), and should be *sui generis*. But serious consideration of the history of religions and, more specifically, postural yoga's
ontological and axiological dimensions, which are reinforced by narrative
traditions and acted out by ritual ones, reveals the problematic nature of
these assumptions.

The Coexistence of Sacred and Profane Attributes

One reason for ignoring the religious dimensions of postural yoga is the so-called superficial, profane, or mundane nature of its goals—postural yoga is said to aim at mere "fitness and health" (Feuerstein 2003) or "exercise and stress-relief" (Carrette and King: 2005: 119).[10]

However, the assumption that one should reject something as a body of religious practice because it emphasizes some aspect of the mundane world would require most of what makes up the history of religions to be disqualified from the category *religion*. In short, the coexistence of sacred and mundane qualities is threaded throughout the history of religions.

Mircea Eliade suggests that the sacred is not some unchanging homogenous thing that humans access directly, but rather that it is endlessly heterogeneous and accessed only through *hierophanies* or "manifestations of the sacred," which occur through human interactions with something else—such as a tree, a river, a storm, a symbol, or an icon—specific to a local, historical, social, or cultural context (1996 [1949]). In short, human encounters with things treated as sacred happen through human encounters with things also treated as mundane.

In fact, anything mundane can become a hierophany. Eliade points to a variety of examples from sacred vegetation (the Indian *soma* or the Iranian *haoma*) to sacred incarnations (the Hindu notion of the *avatara* or divine "descent" into the world as an animal or human or the Christian doctrine of the incarnation of God the father in the son, Jesus). An object's sacred qualities, according to Eliade, are differentiated from its mundane ones, yet its mundane attributes remain unchanged. According to Eliade, "In a hierophany, there exists a paradox because every hierophany whatever…shows, makes manifest, the co-existence of contradictory essences: sacred and profane, spirit and matter, eternal and non-eternal, and so on" (Eliade 1963: 29). He adds: "One must remember the dialectic of the sacred: any object may paradoxically become a hierophany, a receptacle of the sacred, while still participating in its own cosmic environment (a *sacred* stone, e.g., remains nevertheless a *stone* along with other stones)" (1991 [1952]: 84–85).

In the postural yoga context, when B. K. S. Iyengar's students repeat their teacher's famous mantra—"The body is my temple, asanas are my prayers"—or read in one of his monographs—"Health is religious. Ill-health is irreligious" (Iyengar 1988: 10)—they testify to a hierophany, an experience of the mundane flesh, bones, and physical movements and even accoutrement as sacred. Yet a sacred body nevertheless remains a body of flesh and bone, and a sacred yoga mat nevertheless remains a rubber mat.

Postural yoga systems also share a particular ontological perspective on the coexistence of sacred and profane attributes. A nondualist metaphysics—a denial of the fundamental difference between the material world and the sacred world—characterizes postural yoga culture as well as the New Age movement and pop culture spirituality generally. The increasing presence and size of "mind, body, and spirit" sections of global corporate bookstores testify to the preponderance of this metaphysical vision in consumer culture at large. In fact, Hugh B. Urban suggests a nondualist metaphysics is the dominant ontology of consumer culture (Urban 2000; Urban 2003). He suggests that what the New Age movement shares with consumer culture can be found in tantra, the preeminent South Asian model of nondualism (Urban 2000: 270; see also Urban 2003). Urban adds that tantra may be "the very essence of the liberated, holistic spirituality that characterizes the New Age as a whole—a spirituality that would no longer repress the human body, sexuality, and the desire for material prosperity but integrate them with the need for spiritual nourishment" (Urban 2000: 270). Using Fredric Jameson's expression, "the spiritual logic of late capitalism," Urban adds:

> With its apparent union of spirituality and sexuality, sacred transcendence and material enjoyment, Tantrism might well be said to be the ideal religion for late twentieth-century Western consumer culture…"the spiritual logic of late capitalism." (Urban 2000: 270)[11]

Bryan S. Turner adds with regard to this underlying nondualism of consumer culture that, whereas early capitalism featured a subordination of the body to the soul, contemporary capitalist culture treats both as components of the self (1997: 33).

New Age systems also have a long history of a commitment to a nondualist metaphysics and a concomitant concern with enhancing the body as part of self-development (Albanese 2007: 372). In other words, what we find in tantra, we also find in the New Age movement *and* consumer culture, and thus all three coexist quite nicely.[12] Consequently, the New Age and tantra are useful comparative categories for evaluating postural yoga, which also undergoes popularization in contemporary consumer culture because, as noted in Chapters Three and Four, it represents modern yoga's acclimation to that culture.

There is not, in contrast to Carrette and King's suggestion, an absence of "religio-philosophical" qualities in postural yoga. Rather, postural yoga reflects the dominant religio-philosophical mode of consumer culture, which links the self to the body so that the attainment of health and beauty is central to the transformative and transcendent process of self-development. The postural yogi believes herself or himself to transform the body into a temple, a sacred vessel, transcending the mundane flesh and bones while remaining in those very same flesh and bones.

Carrette and King or Feuerstein might retort that "fitness," "stress-relief," and "health" are the "final objectives" of postural yoga and serve utilitarian self-interest as opposed to salvation or other transcendent religious aims. Yet a full understanding of the religious nature of postural yoga's aims requires reflection on the human tendency to seek resolutions to the problems of weakness and suffering. Commenting on New Age healing systems, Wouter J. Hanegraaff suggests they are not concerned only with utilitarian aims of physical and psychological healing but also with the religious problem of human weakness and suffering (1998: 44).[13] Hanegraaff explains:

> In a general sense, "personal growth" can be understood as the shape "religious salvation" takes in the New Age movement: it is affirmed that deliverance from human suffering and weakness will be reached by developing our human potential, which results in our increasingly getting in touch with our inner divinity. Considering the general affinity between salvation and healing, the close connection between personal growth and healing in the New Age Movement is hardly surprising in itself. It is important to note however, that therapy and religious "salvation" tend to merge to an extent perhaps unprecedented in other traditions. (1998: 46)

So therapeutic approaches to healing, such as postural yoga, can play the same role as religious approaches to salvation. In turn, "religious salvation in fact amounts to a radical form of 'healing'" (Hanegraaff 1998: 44).

Many emic accounts of postural yoga evidence that it functions to resolve the problem of suffering and weakness for those who embrace it. Consider preksha dhyana, the Jain hybrid of soteriological yoga and postural yoga discussed in Chapter Three. The samanis, the mendicant teachers of preksha dhyana, commonly describe the goal of yoga as "to understand the true cause of one's misery." This sentiment is distinct from the traditional Jain notion that the world is inherently characterized by violence and thus suffering and the only way to escape the suffering of the world is ascetic withdrawal from it. In postural yoga classes, the samanis teach that at least some of the suffering of the world is avoidable, and avoiding it is the goal of physical yoga practice.

The samanis, like postural yoga teachers generally, often address the everyday problems and concerns of their yoga students, such as body aches or chronic health problems. Unlike postural yoga teachers generally, they maintain that preksha dhyana is characteristically Jain insofar as the goal is "inner purity" and the ultimate aim is realization of the true self as pure soul.[14] Yet the goal of realizing the soul-self is marginal to that of the healthy-self, as indicated by an invitation consistently found on JVB pamphlets and websites: "Let's achieve good health, peace of mind and divine experience without any barrier of caste, creed, sex, race or faith" (see, e.g., JVB Houston 2011). The invitation mentions "good health" first, and the overall message is that preksha dhyana is a means to overcoming physical and psychological suffering as well as achieving "divine experience," which is not defined but instead left open to individual interpretation.

Now consider the Prison Yoga Project. In 2002, James Fox, postural yoga teacher and founder and director of the Prison Yoga Project, began teaching yoga to prisoners at the San Quentin State Prison, a California prison for men (Fig. 5.1). According to the Prison Yoga Project, most prisoners suffer from "original pain," pain caused by chronic trauma experienced early in life (Prison Yoga Project 2008–2010). The consequent suffering leads to violence and thus more suffering in a vicious cycle that can last a lifetime:

> These experiences, imprinted by the terrifying emotions that accompany them, are held deeply in the mind, and perhaps more importantly, in the body, with the dissociative effects of impulsive/reactive behavior, and tendencies toward drug and alcohol addiction as well as violence. Carrying unresolved trauma into their lives impacts everything they do, often landing them in prison, where they experience even more trauma. (Prison Yoga Project 2008–2010)

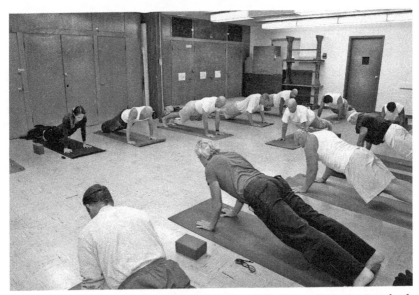

FIGURE 5.1 James Fox, Founder and Director of the Prison Yoga Project, leads students through the *uttihita chaturanga danda asana* (plank posture) in 2012 at San Quentin State Prison in San Quentin, California. Photographed by Robert Sturman. (Courtesy of Robert Sturman.)

Yoga, according to the Prison Yoga Project, provides prisoners dealing with original pain with a path toward healing and recovery as it "is very effective in releasing deeply held, unresolved trauma" (Prison Yoga Project 2008–2010). Yoga is believed to have "transformational, rehabilitative value" for the prisoners and to prevent them from doing more self-harm; it is also believed to increase compassion for others (Prison Yoga Project 2008–2010). Yoga, in short, is an ethical practice meant to prevent more suffering:

> We consistently teach a practice to provide prisoners with a skill to become more sensitive to how they feel in their bodies. When you develop a close relationship with your own sensitivity, you are less apt to violate another. This is empathy. And empathy, when encouraged, leads to compassion. Gradually, the cycle of violence is interrupted. (Prison Yoga Project 2008–2010)

Fox's use of yoga to heal the suffering of at-risk populations is not unprecedented: He learned much of what he applies in the Prison Yoga Project while studying with Joseph H. Pereira, an Iyengar Yoga teacher, Catholic priest, and Founder and Managing Trustee of the Kripa Foundation in India (Kripa Foundation 2006–2007). Founded in 1981, the Kripa Foundation now operates over thirty recovery centers for people with alcohol or drug addiction as well as support centers for people with HIV and AIDS (Kripa Foundation 2009–2010). Pereira is deeply involved with the Ramamani Iyengar Yoga Institute (RIMYI), where he studied yoga extensively with Iyengar and became certified as an Iyengar Yoga teacher (Kripa Foundation 2009–2010). Iyengar Yoga plays a central role in the "holistic component" of the Kripa Foundation's recovery and support programs (Kripa Foundation 2006–2007).

In postural yoga contexts, yogis aim to surmount some types of suffering, but other types of suffering, which involve the disciplining of desire for the sake of body enhancement and healing, are worth pursuing. At first glance, this seems unlikely since postural yoga is a product of a consumer culture in which consumers choose products and services based on individual desires and needs. Consumption of this kind appears rather hedonistic or perhaps, as Carrette and King put it, is characterized by an "*obsession* with the individual self and a distinct lack of interest in compassion, the disciplining of desire, self-less service to others and questions of social justice" (2005: 114).

Mike Featherstone, however, provides a more nuanced analysis of consumer culture, arguing against the common assumption that consumer culture is equivalent to hedonistic consumerism and suggesting instead that a "calculating hedonism," with its own ascetic qualities, characterizes consumer culture (1991: 171). In short, consumer culture facilitates choice with regard to a variety of products and services, but the disciplining of desire and choice-based consumption are not incompatible (1991: 171; see also Turner, Bryan S. 1997: 39).

Global trends in consumer culture at times betray a strong ascetic tone. Whether watching television in Copenhagen or New York, Mumbai or Amsterdam, most commercials target consumers who are assumed to be inadequate and unhappy because they are overweight, lack sex appeal or cannot adequately sexually perform, or are addicted to unhealthy foods or behaviors. Self-development, with the unattainable yet ever-present goal of self-actualization, becoming perfect, is of ultimate value.

Self-development requires a rigorous disciplining of desire because desire puts one at risk for self-destructive, unhealthy habits. The consumer seeks to conquer unhealthy desire in an attempt to cultivate a better self and to live a better life. She fears her consumer choices may otherwise perpetuate imperfection. Tempted by unhealthy desires, the consumer considers purchasing the chocolate candy bar but is reminded of that religious mantra of consumer culture, "You are what you eat," and reaches instead for the organic, whole-grain granola bar.

Today this disciplining of desire finds expression in various ascetic areas of pop culture, from CrossFit, a rigorous fitness regimen advertised as "a program that will best prepare trainees for any physical contingency—not only for the unknown, but for the unknowable" (CrossFit 2013), to Kashi, a whole-grain food company, whose website states, "We think getting healthy starts with taking little steps, like choosing healthy all natural foods. Kashi is about embracing and living your best life" (Kashi Company 2013).

Postural yoga serves as one more way to self-actualize and repent for the modern sins of eating too much sugar, smoking cigarettes, or sitting around watching television. The kinds of asceticism prevalent in postural yoga contexts are not unlike those in traditional religious contexts. Postural yoga is for self-development—most frequently defined in terms of modern conceptions of weight loss, sexual appeal and performance, or health—not for play or pleasure. In postural yoga, pain is put in service of physical and psychological healing and advancement, steps on the path toward perfection.

Consider the "no pain, no gain" mentality that dominates some popular postural yoga systems. One student describes a not uncommon experience in a Bikram Yoga class led by Bikram Choudhury himself:

Before I can do the Head-to-Knee Pose...I have to wipe the sweat out of my eyes and dry my hands and foot to stop them from slipping. Even so, I topple over immediately. I look around. A few of the students can hold the poses until the bitter end, but most, like me, are tortured and teetering while Bikram urges us on, admonishing us to work harder, stretch harder. "Pain is good. You Americans taught me, no pain no gain. In India we say, No hell, no heaven." (Despres n. d.)

On the topic of disciplining desire in the context of consumer culture, Featherstone adds, although asceticism has been invoked throughout religious history in an attempt to liberate the soul from the body, particularly the sexual body, consumer culture features ascetic regimens of diet and exercise aimed at the enhancement of sexual prowess (1991: 182). Postural yoga is no exception.

The Jain samanis embody a paradox here insofar as they lead postural yoga classes in white cotton saris covering most of their bodies, their heads shaved, physically representing the traditional Jain ascetic concern with inverting sexual prowess, yet they lead a class of female consumers concerned with improving their physical appearance and thus enhancing their sexual prowess.[15] In more popular yoga advertisements and publications, women and men are continuously and explicitly invited to embrace a rigorous postural yoga regimen for the sake of attaining the envied "sexy yoga butt."[16] And yoga is not just prescribed as a means to a sexier body, it is also prescribed as a means to better sexual skills. In one yoga class, for example, Choudhury demonstrated the Eagle Pose and explained: "[This pose is] good for sex. Cootchi, cootchi. You can make love for hours and have seven orgasms when you are 90" (Despres n. d.).

Turner contributes an additional insight into the role of the disciplining of desire in consumer culture when he articulates the cultural shift toward the "medicalization of the body in which religious notions of asceticism were gradually replaced by secular medical perspectives and regimens"; this process, Turner suggests, is linked to the "secularization of the body" (1997: 35). Authority with regard to how to discipline desire shifts in the modern context from traditional religious institutions to the biomedical profession, and in response individuals and organizations, including proponents of postural yoga, appropriate biomedical discourse in order to claim that authority. In other words, the religious is not "replaced" by the secular as Turner suggests, but individuals and organizations do seek to manage the body in ways considered compatible with biomedical perspectives on the body.

Preksha dhyana serves as an explicit example of the shift in authority with regard to disciplining desire. The samanis, for example, prescribe an ascetic regimen, including a Jain vegetarian diet, fasting, and postural exercises. Such practices are prescribed for reasons more compatible with the modern consumer context, namely for perceived health benefits, instead of the purification benefits traditionally attributed to them. For example, the samanis most frequently prescribe vegetarianism not for spiritual purification from karma, but because of the connection between the overconsumption of cholesterol-rich meat and heart disease.

The immense market for books on yoga anatomy and physiology, featuring titles such as *Yoga Anatomy*, *The Key Muscles of Yoga: Scientific Keys*, and *Anatomy of Hatha Yoga*, testify to the dominance of biomedical discourse for explaining the benefits of postural yoga. Contorting the body into onerous yoga postures requires years of work disciplining desire for ends explained through biomedical discourse. Iyengar's *Light on Yoga* (1966), a global standard reference on postural yoga, details the anatomical and physiological dimensions of each posture and its health benefits using biomedical discourse. Consider, for example, how Iyengar explains the "effects" of the very difficult *mayura asana* or "peacock posture," in which, facing the floor, the yogi uses her hands to lift the entire body off the ground and holds it as far off the ground as the distance between the wrist and elbow, in a horizontal position:

> This āsana tones the abdominal region of the body, because due to the pressure of the elbows against the abdominal aorta, blood circulates properly in the abdominal organs. This improves digestive power and prevents the accumulation of toxins in the system. It develops and strengthens the elbows, forearms and wrists. (Iyengar 1966: 284)

Since *Light on Yoga's* publication, books on yoga anatomy and physiology have increasingly relied on biomedical terminology and explanations. Leslie Kaminoff and Amy Matthews, authors of the most popular reference on the anatomy and physiology of yoga today, *Yoga Anatomy* (2012), introduce the reader to yoga with four chapters on the human respiratory system (Chapter 1), spine (Chapter 2), skeletal system (Chapter 3), and muscular system (Chapter 4). And all of this before even getting to yoga postures, which are indexed based on the joint or muscle that benefits from each posture. Consider now the description of the effects of the mayura asana in *Yoga Anatomy*:

> As in other bird poses (eagle, crow, rooster, etc.), [mayura asana] involves flexion of the thoracic spine, abduction of the scapulae, and extension of the cervical spine. It's unusual to balance on the arms with the forearms supinated. This changes the action in the elbows, and brings the biceps brachii much more into use. (Kaminoff and Matthews 2012: 239)

The ascetic dimensions of postural yoga also have ritual dimensions. I use *ritual* here in the sense of a set of behaviors that invoke or orient the practitioner toward what is deemed sacred, that which is perceived as transcending conventional life and is therefore somehow set apart or

special. In many premodern systems, yoga was characterized by an initiatory structure whereby the practitioner experienced death to the profane
human condition, which required the practitioner to renounce everything
that seemed important on the conventional level, and rebirth to a sanc-
tified, transcendent modality (Eliade 1990 [1958]: 362–363). Many yoga
practitioners were not renouncers, but the "reversal" of conventional
behavior set renouncer yoga practitioners outside of day-to-day life (Eliade
1990 [1958]: 362) to be reborn into a life characterized by the acquisition of
immortality or "absolute freedom" from conventional limits on consciousness or even the body (Eliade 1990 [1958]: 363–364).

In very different ways, postural yoga also features an initiatory ritual
structure. Citing Arnold van Gennep on rites of passage, Elizabeth de
Michelis argues that a postural yoga class functions as a "healing ritual
of secular religion" (de Michelis 2004: 252).[17] Also citing Victor Turner,
de Michelis argues that the postural yoga class functions as a "liminal
space": "Spatially, practitioners remove themselves from the hustle and
bustle of everyday life to attend the yoga class in a designated 'neutral' (and ideally somewhat secluded) place" (de Michelis 2004: 252).[18]
The practitioner undergoes both physical and psychological transformations and healing before being reintroduced to "everyday life" (de
Michelis 2004: 252–257).

The "liminal space" of the postural yoga class is a space set apart from
the stresses of everyday life (de Michelis 2004), but it does not represent a
renunciation of the profane or conventional life. Rather, the postural yoga
class functions as a space in which to undergo physical and psychological
healing and transformation so that the practitioner can be reintroduced
to everyday life in what is believed to be an improved state. Postural yoga
differs dramatically from the disciplined and systematic techniques for
training and controlling the mind and body that belonged to elite groups
of South Asian renouncers who were concerned with "absolute freedom"
with regard to mortality or consciousness. Postural yoga is, rather, as
Sarah Strauss suggests, a transnational and sometimes socially critical
practice aiming toward "freedom to achieve personal well-being" (Strauss
2005: 22).

Preksha dhyana camps function as an example of yoga's ritual structure. The samanis offer camps in cities where JVB centers are found,
and such camps function to improve overall health by removing practitioners from the stressful life of everyday work and play and immersing
them in a setting where yoga and its concomitant practices, including a

Jain vegetarian diet and abstinence from normal daily activities, followed by reintroduction of the now more health-conscious practitioner back into normal hectic life. A 2007 issue of the JVB newsletter in Houston described an event during a camp that succinctly demonstrates a concern with health. According to the newsletter, a doctor conducted tests and analyses of the blood pressure, sugar, BMI, and body fat of all attendees, including the samanis. The results showed how the samanis' "living style provided a healthy balance" for physical health (Jain Vishva Bharati Houston Newsletter 2007).

The excesses of yoga—retreats, workshops, dieting, onerous postures—signify its reversal of conventional life for the sake of rebirth back into that life as a renewed and better self. And improvement is tracked primarily through biomedical measures.

A problem, according to Carrette and King, with the commodification of a traditional religious product in the context of consumer culture is that "the corporate machine or the market does not seek to validate or reinscribe the tradition but rather utilizes its cultural cachet for its own purposes and profit" (2005: 16). Narrative evidence suggests, however, that "validating" and "reinscribing" yoga are exactly what proponents of postural yoga do by means of appealing to biomedical discourse and by concomitantly locating sacred qualities in the mundane world. In particular, by claiming ancient origins of what are considered biomedically legitimized systems of practice, marketers respond to new cultural desires and demands with products perceived to be both authentically ancient and progressively modern.

There is no doubt that, for many yoga teachers, the claim to possess knowledge of yoga that can be rooted in ancient origins is closely related to their quest for power, status, or money. Some popular books in the yoga market testify to the common goal among yoga entrepreneurs of teaching yoga while making a profit. Two examples are *Selling Yoga: A Handbook for the Ultimate Yoga Business Professional* (2008) by Ron Thatcher and *The Yogi Entrepreneur: A Guide to Earning a Mindful Living through Yoga* (2011) by Darren Main. Excerpts from the back cover of Thatcher's book include "*Selling Yoga* is an income-producing system"; "It's one thing to be able to teach innovative and exotic classes, but to become powerful and successful with your own business in yoga is the ultimate goal and what you will learn in this book"; and "Ron Thatcher has a proven track record as a top producer in the Yoga and Fitness industry...Thousands of sales professionals and managers have used his techniques to improve their paychecks" (Thatcher 2008). And here is an excerpt from the back cover of Main's *The Yogi Entrepreneur*: "With more than fifty free and low-cost marketing tips and dozens of resources, this book will help teachers world-wide realize that balancing your checkbook can be every bit as yogic as doing a headstand" (Main 2011).

There is, however, much more to the business of postural yoga than who profits. The claim to authority with regard to ancient yoga knowledge serves to ground a worldview and set of values and therefore fulfills a mythological function.[19] Mara Einstein suggests that mythologizing is at work in branding, which requires marketers to uniquely package their products (Einstein 2008: 12).

Postural yoga giants Iyengar and K. Pattabhi Jois serve as exempla of how branding and mythologizing go hand in hand. Both mythologize their systems of postural yoga in ways that tie those systems to ancient yoga traditions while simultaneously reflecting dominant cultural ideas and values by claiming biomedical authority. Their myths ground postural yoga in a linear trajectory of transmission—premodern yoga functions as what Mark Singleton describes as "the touchstone of authenticity" for proponents of modern yoga (Singleton 2010:14). Claims to that transmission are frequently made and assumed to be historically accurate. While Iyengar has historically claimed ties between Iyengar Yoga and the ancient yoga transmission going at least as far back as the *Yoga Sutras*, as discussed in Chapter Four, he recently introduced a ritual invocation to Patanjali at the beginning of each Iyengar Yoga class in order to further associate his yoga system with that transmission. Iyengar also presents yoga as biomedically legitimized, as is evidenced by the biomedical discourse that permeates his work on yoga, referring, for example, to the asanas' benefits for "every muscle, nerve and gland in the body" (Iyengar 1966: 40).

In like manner, Jois suggested that verses from the earliest Vedas delineate the nine postures of the *surya namaskar* sequences of postures in his Ashtanga Vinyasa yoga system (Singleton 2010: 221–222, n. 4).[20] He also reevaluates the purification function of yoga as resulting not in the purification from karma, but in the purification from disease:

> The purpose of *vinyasa* is for internal cleansing. Breathing and moving together while performing *asanas* makes the blood hot, or as Pattabhi Jois says, boils the blood. Thick blood is dirty and

causes disease in the body. The heat created from yoga cleans the blood and makes it thin, so that it may circulate freely. The combination of the *asanas* with movement and breath make the blood circulate freely around all the joints, taking away body pains. When there is a lack of circulation, pain occurs. The heated blood also moves through all the internal organs removing impurities and disease, which are brought out of the body by the sweat that occurs during practice. (Shri K. Pattabhi Jois Ashtanga Yoga Institute 2009)

In the postural yoga world, branding and mythologizing simultaneously involve validating yoga based on its ties to both ancient origins and modern science.

The (Non)Ethics of Religious Practice

Postural yoga is, in part, a product of consumer culture, which emerged out of the socioeconomic complex of global market capitalism. That there are ethical problems with market capitalism, given its dire consequences for individuals, communities, and the natural environment, is indisputable. Carrette and King understandably are concerned about the "pernicious social effects of neoliberalism and the corporate takeover of society," namely the displacement of "questions of social justice" (Carrette and King 2005: x). The ethical implications of market capitalism in the light of modern commitments to the individual (or human rights), the social world (or social justice), and the natural environment (or sustainability) are dire. In other words, if one's ethical agenda is a modern one that includes maintaining a stable global community of equal persons and a sustainable natural environment, market capitalism is rightfully perceived as an obstacle.

That the ethical problems with market capitalism make the products of consumer culture, by definition, nonreligious, however, is disputable. Carrette and King's reduction of pop culture spiritualities to the mere commodification of what were traditional religious wares frames spirituality as distinct from religion and presumes, therefore, that spirituality cannot itself function as a body of religious practice. As a product of consumer culture and, therefore, a reflection of capitalist values, postural yoga serves to *replace* religion, not to fulfill religious functions itself. In short, Carrette and King equate the good or ethical with the religious.

Carrette and King problematically and anachronistically read a selfless ethical agenda based on a modern notion of social justice into the so-called religious ancient yoga systems (2005: 116). They then contrast ancient yoga with modern postural yoga, arguing that modern postural yoga pacifies and accommodates consumers who are perpetually motivated to act by their self-interests, not by social justice (2005: 119–121). Finally, they contrast ancient yoga with postural yoga, which serves instead to pacify and accommodate individuals who, as consumers, are perpetually motivated to act in service to their own self-interest (2005: 119–121).

One could easily dispute the assumptions that ethical values are absent in postural yoga by pointing to examples of individuals or organizations that explicitly attach an ethical dimension to yoga practice. Examples discussed above include the Prison Yoga Project and the Kripa Foundation. But that still leaves the majority of the postural yoga world, made up of for-profit companies, unaccounted for.

Yet one would be mistaken to take an ethical agenda as a necessary condition for what type of yoga should be taken seriously as a body of religious practice. Evidence suggests that premodern yoga systems, though religious, were not ethical in any modern sense. And an assessment of postural yoga that does not take it seriously as a body of religious practice on account of its lack of an essential moral code, even if such an assessment left room for exceptions, would be far too simplistic.

First, critical scholarship on the history of religions does not take ethical as a necessary condition for something to qualify as religious. Consider the etymology of some of the most dominant categories in the study of religion: *sacred* and *holy*. In *The Elementary Forms of Religious Life* (1912), Émile Durkheim famously uses the term *sacred* in his definition of religion: "a unified system of beliefs and practices relative to sacred things, that is to say, things set apart and forbidden—beliefs and practices which unite into one single moral community called a Church, all those who adhere to them" (2001 [1912]: 62). The sacred, in short, is that which is set apart from the ordinary or profane. This meaning of *sacred* is evident in the etymology of the term, which can be traced back to the Latin terms *sacer, sacrum*, and *sanctum*. In Roman society, the *sacrum*, on the one hand, belonged to the gods or a god and was present in the *sanctum* or interior space of a temple. The *profanum* or "profane," on the other hand, was "in front of" (*pro-*) the "temple" (*fanum*) and therefore outside the *sanctum* or sacred interior space of a temple.

Focusing more on religious experience, Rudolf Otto, in *The Idea of the Holy* (1917), famously defined the sacred or "the holy" as the human experience of a *mysterium tremendum et fascinans*—that is, a mystical presence (*mysterium*) simultaneously terrifying (*tremendum*) and alluring (*fascinans*). Otto explains:

> The fact is we have come to use the words "holy," "sacred" [heilig], in an entirely derivative sense, quite different from that which they originally bore. We generally take "holy" as meaning "completely good"...But this common usage of the term is inaccurate. It is true that all this moral significance is contained in the word "holy," but it includes in addition—as even as we cannot but feel—a clear overplus of meaning, and this it is now our task to isolate. Nor is this merely a later or acquired meaning; rather, "holy," or at least the equivalent words in Latin and Greek, in Semitic and other ancient languages, denoted first and foremost *only* this overplus: if the ethical element was present at all, at any rate it was not original and never constituted the whole meaning of the word. (Otto 1958 [1917]: 5)

In short, what is sacred (or holy) is not necessarily good; the sacred, rather, is sacred.

Experiences of or behaviors based on what is sacred—Eliade, as noted above, suggests these occur in and through the mundane—are neither ethical in themselves, nor do they always lead to ethical action. Some of religious history's most transformative and ethical moments as well as some of its most horrible and violent ones have been instigated or supported by what was believed to be or treated as sacred.

Take, as a modern example, the life of the Indian guru Sathya Sai Baba (1926–2011) (Fig. 5.2).[21] Reflecting on Sai Baba's life, one encounters moments of divine transformation, devotion, and social service as well as pain, death, and heinous accusations. Millions of devotees believed in and worshiped Sai Baba as a *godman*. Many also despised him as a charlatan, a sexual abuser, and even an accessory to murder.

In 1963, Sai Baba disclosed that he was the incarnation of God himself, a God that transcends all religious boundaries. His ecumenical teaching maintained that all religions are true paths to God, and since Sai Baba was God, he was also Shiva, Vishnu, Jesus, and Allah. Sai Baba's ability to attract devotees—whether attributed to his personal charisma,

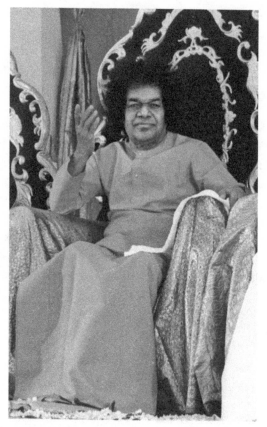

FIGURE 5.2 Sai Baba in 1996 at his Brindavan ashram in Bangalore. Photographed by Guy Veloso. Licensed under the Creative Commons Attribution-Share Alike 3.0 Unported license. Accessed through Wikimedia Commons.

marketing skills, or both—was extraordinary. Today the International Sathya Sai Organization disseminates Sai Baba's teachings and manages a network of over twelve hundred Sathya Sai Baba centers in over one hundred countries. Most of his devotees acknowledged him as divine without ever meeting him in person.

As Sai Baba's devotees grew in numbers and influence, so did his financial worth. In 1972 the Sathya Sai Central Trust was established; today it is estimated to be worth at least $8.9 billion. It has funded water supply projects in poor areas of southern India as well as ashrams, hospitals, universities, and several schools across India and globally.

Sai Baba was most famous for his miracles—mainly materializations of valuable objects. The guru was believed to miraculously heal the sick and to leave his body in order to visit people across the world. For devotees, such miracles confirmed that Sai Baba was God incarnate.

Others disagreed. Sai Baba's reputation was tinged by accusations that he was a charlatan. Skeptics argued that his abilities were simply the sign of a skilled conjuring magician. Perhaps the most notable controversy surrounding the guru arose in 1993 when the police killed six young male devotees in Sai Baba's bedroom and claimed that they did so in self-defense. Some speculate that the men were not killed in self-defense but were murdered after they arrived to confront Sai Baba or perhaps kill him in retribution.

In retribution for what? There were accusations that Sai Baba sexually abused some of his male devotees. Such accusations received global attention when in 2004 the British Broadcasting Corporation (BBC) aired *Secret Swami*, a documentary featuring interviews with American devotees who claimed Sai Baba had coerced them as young men into sexual relationships. They described how he initiated them into such relationships by rubbing oil on their genitals and then proceeded to demand sexual favors, in some cases for years. Sai Baba denied the allegations and was never officially investigated nor charged with any crime in India.

Sai Baba's life was a complex one to say the least, and it calls into question how we use the term *guru*. Terms for religious exempla, such as *saint* or *guru*, generally occur in the popular imagination in reference to figures assumed to be sacred (or to have special access to what is sacred) and to be ethically virtuous. But how could Sai Baba, a global guru loved by many and simultaneously marred by controversy, have been *both* a religious exemplar as guru and godman and an abuser, a cheat, or an accessory to murder? On the one hand, devotees claim that their charitable service to less fortunate communities is substantial and is a direct consequence of Sai Baba's teachings and transformative effects in their lives. And money from the Sathya Sai Central Trust has been used to improve the lives of hundreds of thousands of people living in poor conditions. On the other hand, accusations that he used fraudulent magic to coerce devotees, threatened devotees to have sex with him, and perhaps even participated as an accessory to murder are impossible to ignore. If any one of these accusations is true it is difficult to consider Sai Baba a *guru*—assuming that religious term has something to do with both what is sacred and what is ethical.

But the history of religions is tinged by religious exempla with questionable ethics. By destabilizing popular assumptions about what qualifies as sacred, it becomes possible to adequately evaluate Sai Baba's life and to bracket—and even denounce—his ethics while still acknowledging the transformative effects he had on his devotees. In this case the religious term *guru* would point not to individuals with exceptional virtue, but to those who represent something sacred, which gives them power to convince, to lead, and to instigate positive transformation. In Sai Baba's case, this much, at least, was true. So there is reason and precedence to dislodge the meaning of sacred from direct associations with ethics.

Take, as an ancient example, the history of premodern yoga. Carrette and King suggest that a selfless ethical agenda in service to society and even the greater cosmos characterizes ancient yoga systems (2005: 116, 119–121). At least all Hindu and Buddhist premodern yoga systems, according to Carrette and King, "share in common" this ethical agenda (2005: 116). Yet an ethical agenda in the modern sense privileged by Carrette and King was never an essential characteristic of yoga. Rather, premodern yoga can be, as Eliade put it, both antisocial and antihuman (Eliade 1990 [1958]: 95).

In premodern traditions, yoga functions on its own ethical terms, in a sense specific to each system's time and place, as a religious complex of "disciplined and systematic techniques for the training and control of the human mind-body complex, which are also understood as techniques for the reshaping of human consciousness towards some kind of higher goal" (Samuel 2008: 2). Many premodern yoga systems are believed to instigate transformative and transcendent states that scholars have described as sacred, yet they require the adept to be removed from structures that render social ethics of any sort possible.[22] In many premodern yoga systems, such as Patanjala or Jain yoga, the practitioner is an ascetic to the extent that he or she is removed from the relational webs of conventional society, intentional action, and the natural environment, with the practitioner's own body regarded as the most intimate expression of that environment. The ascetic dimensions of yoga conflict with the attribution of intrinsic value to the body—an attribution that is, necessarily, concomitant with human life and is a necessary condition for active and restorative engagement with human suffering. It is because of their general hostility to the conventional and natural worlds and all they entail that many premodern yoga systems are not ethical in any modern sense of the term. Like Christian or Jewish mystics, premodern yoga practitioners may have claimed to have direct access to God or the divine, but they nevertheless do not speak to modern concerns about social or environmental ethics.

The basic point is that, to the extent that yoga is ascetic and world-denying, it is ethically problematic for anyone whose first concern is with physical suffering, social justice, or the natural environment—likewise to the extent that yoga perpetuates market capitalism. Not all yoga systems, despite their status as bodies of religious practice, can help us with our contemporary ethical tasks, unless we are willing to abandon specifically modern conceptions of what ethics *is*. The categorical distinction between what is sacred and good or ethical frees us to criticize yoga systems, whether premodern or modern, from a modern ethical perspective, while at the same time appreciating them as bodies of religious practice.

The Religious Is Not Sui Generis

In an attempt to write off postural yoga as a body of religious practice, Carrette and King reduce it to nothing more than a commodity of consumer culture. In contrast, in an attempt to argue on behalf of taking premodern yoga seriously as a body of religious practice, they presume its *sui generis* nature and ossified ethical center or essence. The juxtaposition of a noncontextualized premodern yoga tradition against a contextualized postural yoga one is problematic. Invoking the context-sensitive nature of postural yoga and contrasting it with the supposed sui generis nature of premodern yoga in defense of not taking postural yoga seriously as a body of religious practice requires an act of historical reconstruction. Like postural yoga, all premodern yoga systems are situated within social contexts that, in turn, bring about various transformations. As discussed in detail in Chapter One, yoga systems prior to the dominance of market capitalism, in the same way as yoga systems following the dominance of market capitalism, were framed by the values of their respective societies.

Although yoga "retained some of its integrity as a specific set of techniques for self-cultivation through all of these transformations," a full understanding of each system of premodern yoga requires consideration of the "specific context within which it was adopted and transformed" (Samuel 2007: 186). In fact, Vesna Wallace suggests that the environments of premodern yoga systems "became replicated in the structures" of those systems and even "determined their social values" (Wallace 2011: 336). Even if certain social principles of religious complexes were, in theory, socially radical, those principles "can become transformed and in some cases even nullified in response to historical and sociopolitical contexts" (Wallace 2011: 336).

In Chapter One, I cited numerous recent studies (e.g., Davidson 2002; Chapple 2003; White 2006; Bronkhorst 2007; Samuel 2008; White 2009; Chapple 2011; Wallace 2011; Larson 2012; White 2012) that attend to the particularities of premodern yoga systems, which vary based largely on social context. These studies resist misrepresentations of premodern yoga as timeless and homogenous. In short, their discussions based on empirical data suggest that premodern yoga systems, made up of a heterogeneous mix of complex ritual, ideological, and narrative traditions, never appear outside of social contexts.

Furthermore, refusals to take modern postural yoga seriously as a body of religious practice based on the argument that it is a product of global market capitalism ignores historical evidence suggesting that postural yoga emerged out of a much longer religious history (see, e.g., Hanegraaff 1998; de Michelis 2005; Albanese 2007; Singleton 2010). In fact, Catherine Albanese places both the New Age movement and modern yoga along the same historical trajectory of what she terms "metaphysical religion" in Britain and the United States, the earliest precursors of which go as far back as Hellenic and Hermetic thought (2007). As discussed in Chapter Two, that history can be traced up through the nineteenth- and early-twentieth-century Romantic and Orientalist appropriations of the "East" (Albanese 2007).

It is certainly the case that, by means of reform and innovation, modern yoga proponents constructed new approaches to premodern South Asian yoga systems and thus reevaluated certain ancient categories. Some of the key elements in the process of constructing postural yoga discussed in preceding chapters included a disassociation from the negative stereotypes associated with the so-called extreme ascetic practices that Orientalists and colonialists equated with hatha yoga, the appropriation of biomedical discourse and practices dominant in the global fitness market, a concern with the enhancement of the body according to modern standards, and a modern pluralist outlook that requires no formal religious affiliation or identity.

Processes of assimilation and adaptation, however, are characteristic of the history of religions and, more specifically, the history of yoga both before and within the context of global market capitalism, and thus we cannot equate such processes with capitalist commodity exchange. Since

Carrette and King's criticism of the borrowing and reconstructing that is characteristic of postural yoga is in fact characteristic of the history of yoga generally, readers are left to consider whether or not there is something unique to the context of consumer culture that excludes its products from the category of *religion*. Indeed, Carrette and King's analysis focuses not on the claim that postural yoga arises from a social context, but that it arises solely from the social context dominant in the age of global capitalism. They are troubled by the fact that a particular socioeconomic complex—that is, market capitalism—has influenced the production and marketing of postural yoga.

Yet, as a variety of thinkers suggest, although the commodities of consumer culture are manifestations of it, it would be a mistake to reduce consumer culture to those commodities (Featherstone 1991; Bocock 1993; Tomlinson 1999: 83). With regard to consumer culture, Featherstone argues, not only are there immaterial objects of consumption, but also new cultural products are not always "fed through the commodity market process" (Featherstone 2007: xxiii.). Featherstone explains:

> ...modernity with its processes of rationalization, commodification, secularization and disenchantment does not lead to the eclipse of religious sentiments, for while formal religions may decline, symbolic classifications and ritual practices which embody sacred/profane distinctions live on at the heart of secular social processes. As Durkheim pointed out, anything can become sacred, so why not the "profane" goods of capitalism? If we focus on the actual use of commodities it is clear that in certain settings they can become de-commodified and receive a symbolic charge (over and above that intended by the advertisers) which makes them sacred to their users. (Featherstone 2007: 119)

A close evaluation of postural yoga in particular suggests that, although the commodities of yoga brands are manifestations of it, it would be a mistake to reduce yoga to those commodities. In fact, postural yoga as a body of religious practice and commodification are not mutually exclusive; rather, they stand in a symbiotic relationship to one another. The yoga market, in accordance with consumer culture in general (Featherstone 1991: 112; Bocock 1993), destabilizes the basic utility of yoga commodities and services and assigns to them new meanings. In other words, yoga brands, whether they signify a particular teacher, style,

124 SELLING YOGA

or product, signify more than just the fulfillment of utilitarian needs; rather, the fulfillment of religious needs becomes contained in the brand. Put more simply, postural yoga's rituals and narratives reflect yogis' deepest values and most sacred goals.

Often, postural yogis overtly describe the aims of their yoga practice in religious terms. Consider, for example, the TYA, which maintains that yoga is an ancient practice composed of a plurality of branches and that it developed as a "spiritual" and "religious" practice, not simply as a "trade skill" or "sport" (Texas Yoga Association 2011). Also consider the cover of the February 25, 2011, "Belief" section of the *Houston Chronicle*, which featured an image of Buergermeister in fashionable yoga attire and in the posture of a South Asian goddess, complete (thanks to clever photography) with six arms (Shellnutt 2011). Below the image, the headline reads, "THE SOUL OF YOGA" (Shellnutt 2011). For those yogis interviewed in the article, yoga is not a mere profane commodity; it is a deeply transformative, perhaps even divine, tradition. In the article, Buergermeister describes how yoga helped her connect with "God as a creator, as a source" and brought her "closer to my divinity" (Shellnutt 2011: F7). Another postural yogi interviewed for the article, Roger Rippy, a local yoga practitioner, teacher, and studio owner, rejects that yoga is a religion but nonetheless invokes explicitly religious discourse to describe yoga: "Yoga isn't a religion" because "It doesn't give you a dogma"; rather, "it's about your own particular practice and your own particular relationship with God" (Shellnutt 2011: F7).

Though many postural yogis prefer to describe their practice as "spiritual," others eagerly associate the religious dimensions of yoga with specific religious traditions or institutions. It is not unusual to find overt religious packaging of yoga brands. In the history of postural yoga, yoga advocates have packaged yoga in modern metaphysical, scientific, and fitness materials. In the history of premodern and early modern yoga, advocates packaged yoga in everything from Buddhist, Hindu, and Jain materials to Protestant materials. Today, postural yoga continues to be packaged in overtly religious ways to meet the desires of specific consumer audiences. We already witnessed how this occurs in preksha dhyana and Anusara Yoga, in which postural yoga is packaged in modern Jain and modern tantric materials respectively.

But efforts to package postural yoga in overtly religious ways are not limited to cases that draw from South Asian religious discourses. Some contemporary Christians, Jews, and Muslims, in fact, argue that the universal psychological and physical benefits of yoga can be separated from the Hindu, Buddhist, Jain, or other South Asian doctrine-specific expressions and then reconstructed as an essential component of the Christian, Jewish, or Muslim life respectively.

Estelle Eugene, founder and Director of the Jewish Yoga Network in the United Kingdom, suggests yoga can contribute to a well-lived Jewish life. Her organization's website features the following testimony from Rabbi David Rosen:

Whether one sees Yoga as helping recapture Jewish wisdom and practice which may have been lost over time, or as incorporating wisdom from other parts of the world into Jewish life; the physical and spiritual benefits of such practice offer much blessing and enlightenment. (Jewish Yoga Network 2011)

Muslim community activist Muhammad Rashid and Imam Mohd A. Qayyoom have both encouraged Muslims in Queens, New York, to practice yoga and even performed their daily prayers (*salat*) on their yoga mats during an interfaith festival in Jackson Heights, New York. Rashid explains, "I discovered whatever I'm doing in yoga, I'm doing five times a day in prayer" (Nir 2012).

The overt Christianization of yoga occurs on an individual level. For example, one Protestant Christian and yoga practitioner, Agnieszka Tennant, shares the following: "The three hours a week I spend doing yoga not only make me more flexible, tone my muscles, and relax me. They also draw me closer to Christ. They are my bodily-kinetic prayer" (Tennant 2005).[23] The Reverend Anthony Randazzo, a priest at Notre Dame Roman Catholic Church in North Caldwell, New Jersey, has practiced and taught yoga for over ten years and insists that it has always brought him closer to Christ and that he is "more deeply rooted in the Christian faith than ever" (Alvarez 2010).

Christian yoga brands and products or yoga-inspired fitness brands and products that claim to enhance and strengthen the Christian identities of their consumers are also increasingly popular. One Catholic practitioner of yoga, Jean Marie Déchanet, prescribed yoga for Christians and coined the term *Christian Yoga* in her book by that title (1960). Catholic priest Joseph Pereira, mentioned earlier in the chapter, has written or produced several handbooks, CDs, and DVDs that combine his Christian religiosity with yoga, including a handbook and DVD titled *Yoga for the Practice of Christian Meditation*; a video-cassette titled *Living with AIDS*; and a CD titled *The Whole Person in Prayer* (Kripa Foundation 2009–2010). Catholic priest Thomas Ryan is both Director of the North American Paulist Office for Ecumenical and Interfaith Relations and a certified Kripalu Yoga instructor; he created a DVD, *Yoga Prayer: An Embodied Christian Spiritual Practice* (2004), which instructs the audience in how to make yoga a Christian practice. According to Ryan's website, the DVD includes fifty minutes of yoga postures while also teaching how to "pray with your whole body"; it offers "an embodied practice to renew and invigorate your connection to God" and invites its audience to "come home to your body as a temple of the indwelling presence of God" (Paulist Office for Ecumenical and Interfaith Relations).

Many Christians have constructed "Christian" yoga brands, such as Christoga, Yahweh Yoga, and Christ Centered Yoga. In 2003, Brooke Boon founded Holy Yoga, a postural yoga system that functions as "an experiential worship created to deepen people's connection to Christ" (Holy Yoga 2007–2010). Holy Yoga has an Instructor Training Program, and there are currently over three hundred Holy Yoga classes each week in the United States and Canada (Holy Yoga 2007–2010).[24] Such Christian yoga brands often assign Christian terms and prayers to certain yoga postures or sequences and replace South Asian imagery, such as the popular "Om" symbol, with Christian imagery, such as the cross.

Other Christian postural fitness systems, such as WholyFit and PraiseMoves, remove all explicitly yogic language and imagery, including the term *yoga* itself, to avoid what they perceive to be non-Christian associations.[25] Laurette Willis, a public speaker and fitness trainer, promotes PraiseMoves, for example, as "the Christian alternative to yoga" (PraiseMoves 2010).

The extent to which postural yoga that does not have a particular religious affiliation still functions as a body of religious practice is perhaps most obvious in contexts in which yoga consumers do not spend money. In the economic circumstances of market capitalism, the consumption of yoga products and services almost always requires the consumer to spend money, but there are exceptions. The yoga practitioner can now opt out of purchasing a yoga mat altogether or can attend donation-based yoga classes. Such phenomena are becoming especially prevalent in New York City, where organizations offer donation-based yoga classes (the most popular is the hot yoga brand Yoga to the People) or yoga classes that do not require a mat (such as Laughing Lotus, which has studios in New York and San Francisco; Laughing Lotus 2012). Some yogis choose such brands of yoga because those brands are believed to better signify what yogis consider the true "spirit of yoga."

Yoga to the People opened its first studio in 2006 with a donation-only structure. The website bestows the following "mantra":

> There will be no correct clothes
> There will be no proper payment
> There will be no right answers
> No glorified teachers
> No ego no script no pedestals
> No you're not good enough or rich enough
> This yoga is for everyone
> This sweating and breathing and becoming
> This knowing glowing feeling
> Is for the big small weak and strong
> Able and crazy
> Brothers sisters grandmothers
> The mighty and meek
> Bones that creak
> Those who seek
> This power is for everyone. (Yoga to the People 2011b)

In certain ways, Yoga to the People is akin to commodified yoga brands. Consider the benefits Yoga to the People promises: yoga helps people "look and feel great"; "yoga helps tone and sculpt muscles while gaining strength, flexibility and balance"; and "[in] a world of stress, yoga helps people decompress and achieve a sense of inner peace, aiding in healing injury or disease" (Yoga to the People 2011). These are all benefits popularly associated with yoga commodities. Yoga to the People also sells yoga apparel, although the website states:

> Our clothing was not produced with an emphasis on "maximizing" profits. [The] emphasis is to spread the word...to share the intention of YTTP ~ which is to put the essence or spirit of yoga before the business of yoga. (Yoga to the People 2011c)

For the founder of Yoga to the People, Greg Gumucio (a former student of Choudhury's) and those who consume the services associated with his brand, yoga's meaning transcends its commodities.[26] Gumucio states, "I truly believe if more people were doing yoga, the world would be a better place" (Billard 2010a). The anti-commodification brand of Yoga to the People signifies, quite directly, a very particular goal: a better world. That is possible as more and more people become self-actualized or come into their full being—yoga is "becoming"—through strengthening and healing their bodies and minds. The individual who chooses Yoga to the People still acts as a consumer even if consumption does not require the exchange of money. And the consumer chooses Gumucio's brand as opposed to others because of that brand's success in capturing what yoga means to him or her.

Some postural yogis reject the yoga mat for its perceived over-commodification.[27] The mat, for most postural yogis, is a necessity, not just because it allows one to perform postures without slipping or to mark one's territory in a crowded class, but also because it signifies various nonutilitarian meanings. The mat signifies a "liminal space" set apart from day-to-day life as one participates in a self-developmental ritual of rigorous physical practice. It is also often a status symbol. But yogis who reject mats argue that they are not necessary, that they interfere with practice, and that they are simply commodities without any profound meaning. One such yogi argues, "The ecstasy of yoga can't be contained by a mat" (Billard 2010b). Such yogis choose brands of yoga that do not require the mat, such as Laughing Lotus (Laughing Lotus 2012), because those brands are believed to better signify the true meaning of yoga. For the yogi quoted above, that meaning is experiential and transcends ownership of a commodity as seemingly arbitrary as a mat.

Conclusion

Although there is no doubt that many of the ways in which yoga proponents market postural yoga link it to consumer culture, yoga marketers and consumers reflect the fact that not all consumption is the mere consumption of material goods for hedonistic or utilitarian aims. This is evident when one uncovers the religious functions and meanings of postural yoga, not in isolated Indian ashrams, but in pop culture magazines, strip-mall yoga studios, and mainstream websites. Thus, branding products and making them sacred are not incompatible but analogous and compatible processes. In the same way that religious individuals and institutions demarcate what counts as sacred, marketers demarcate a brand by making it special, by setting it apart, which often involves attributing religious functions and meanings to it.

I began this chapter describing the attempts in Texas to regulate yoga and the opposition to such regulation. Regulation of something requires a legal definition of the thing targeted and, like religious institutions and organizations, yoga was assumed to be beyond the reach of a legal definition. Yet the debate over state regulation of yoga in Texas brought questions to light about how one would formulate a legal definition of yoga, if that were even possible. Such an attempt to legally define yoga would amount to identifying a bounded tradition of symbols, practices, and ideas that in reality vary across yoga studios and ashrams within Texas alone. In short, the problem with any legal definition of yoga, whether for the sake of promoting or preventing regulation, is this: Who's to say what is yoga?

For some outsiders to postural yoga, yoga is a mere commodity. But in any serious analysis of postural yoga, privileging only the outsider's perspective results in an account that does not take people's experiences of or desires for yoga seriously. How could it then claim to adequately explain or even describe those experiences or desires? In this chapter, I considered both insider and outsider perspectives on postural yoga and developed an understanding of postural yoga as a body of religious practice.[28]

6

Yogaphobia and Hindu Origins

During the Chicago riots in 1968 where [Allen Ginsberg]
had chanted "Om" for seven hours to calm everyone
down, an Indian gentleman had passed him a note tell-
ing him his pronunciation was all wrong.

—DEBORAH BAKER (2008: 214–215)

IN THE LAST three chapters, I looked closely at popularized yoga, and
I found a lot of spandex-clad, perspiring, toned bodies brought together in
rooms filled with yoga mats and engaged in a sacred fitness regimen set
apart from day-to-day life. In those spaces, Christians, Hindus, atheists,
and others gather to enhance something many of them deem sacred: their
bodies, their selves. These are images never seen before in the history of
yoga—"Do these yogis have it all wrong?"

It turns out that the frequency with which people encounter yoga
today has not translated into an absence of religious protests against it. In
other words, many think these postural yogis do, in fact, have it all wrong.
A growing movement courts fear and suspicion of yoga in its popularized
forms, arguing that people have been duped into thinking that yoga is
simply a product for enhancing physical and psychological well-being.[1]
Protesters target the most popular forms of modern yoga today, those
of postural yoga. The movement warns that yoga, in all of its forms,
is in fact religious and, more specifically, Hindu. For some protesters,
this means that Christians must choose Christianity over yoga lest they
defy Christian doctrine and jeopardize the status of their souls as well
as Christianity's place in the world. For others, this means that postural
yoga can be reduced to a profit-driven market featuring commodities that
corrupt an authentic Hindu system.

This study is suspicious of such protests against the popularization of yoga that rely on definitions of yoga as a homogenous, static Hindu system.[2] Throughout the history of modern yoga there have been many such attempts, and as I write, over a decade into the twenty-first century, I see no sign of them abating. Protesters suggest that yoga has an essential set of characteristics, including that it is Hindu (some recognize it as also Jain, Buddhist, or, more broadly but still essentializing, "Eastern"). From this perspective, yoga belongs within a reified and homogenous tradition, usually the tradition termed *Hinduism*. Hence they criticize those who practice yoga in ways deemed inauthentic and warn them of yoga's Hindu essence. The most suspicious and fear-inciting critics include certain Christians, but such Christians have Hindu bedfellows in defining yoga as Hindu. I call the two positions that emerge from this movement the *Christian yogaphobic position* and the *Hindu origins position*.

On the one hand, advocates of the Christian yogaphobic position warn about the potential dangers of yoga for Christians given the perceived incompatibility between the Hindu essence of yoga and Christian doctrine.[3] They attempt to convince Christians that religious conflict is inevitable if they embrace yoga, given the irreconcilable differences between *them* (i.e., Hindus) and *us* (i.e., Christians). And some American Christians add that yoga's popularization contributes to the establishment of a "post-Christian" nation, something Americans should fear.[4]

On the other hand, advocates of the Hindu origins position criticize postural yogis for failing to recognize yoga's so-called Hindu origins and, in turn, denounce what they consider yoga marketers' illegitimate cooptation and commodification of yoga. Their appeal to origins places them on the ideological trajectory of modern Hindu reformist and nationalist movements insofar as they presume that a narrowly selected list of characteristics are essential to Hinduism and, more specifically, to yoga.

The protests discussed here cannot stand serious historical scrutiny. For most contemporary practitioners of yoga and scholars of religion, yoga is a heterogeneous tradition beyond the scope of rigid definitional boundaries.[5] As articulated by David Gordon White:

Every group in every age has created its own version and vision of yoga. One reason this has been possible is that its semantic field— the range of meanings of the term "yoga"—is so broad and the concept of yoga so malleable, that it has been possible to morph it into nearly any practice or process one chooses. (White 2012: 2)

In this chapter, I critically assess the protests against the popularization of yoga represented by the Christian yogaphobic position and
the Hindu origins position and suggest that these positions are not just
polemical but also prescriptive—that is, they explain how popularized
systems of postural yoga are damaging for a true Christian or Hindu
as well as prescribe narrow visions of how a Christian or Hindu *should*
be religious. In this way, both Christian and Hindu strategies reflect the
prescriptive agenda of religious fundamentalism.[6] Protesters prescribe a
return to what they perceive as the unchanging essence of their respective
religions, which is perceived to have been intact before modernity and,
more specifically, the popularization of postural yoga.

Second, relying on Edward Said's (1978) notion of *Orientalism*, I demonstrate that, although these positions do not serve direct colonial rule,
the regime of knowledge they support perpetuates divisive representations of yoga that fail to account for the realities of living postural yogis
and instead reveal more about protesters' own subjectivity.[7] They function
to alienate Hindus and Christians from each other as well as from perceived others within their own traditions. The Christian yogaphobic position and the Hindu origins position both posit essentialist definitions of
yoga and warnings against its embrace (at least in its popularized forms).
They do so without apparent awareness that such definitions and warnings betray Orientalist strategies, and they fail to recognize that the legitimate historical task is not to search for an authentic form of yoga. In fact,
an authentic form of yoga does not exist.

And finally, I offer a way of moving beyond essentialist conceptions of yoga. Like the essentialist notion of Hinduism, which derived
from Orientalist and Hindu reformist conceptions of religion and have
become a part of academic and popular discourses, essentialist conceptions of yoga threaten to influence both the study and practice of yoga
today.[8] I suggest that we move beyond essentialist conceptions of yoga by
understanding postural yoga and its popularization in terms of the cultural forces that shape its history and development as well as those that
shape the protests against it. Based on that approach, I suggest that the
Christian yogaphobic position and the Hindu origins position emerge
more from the cultural context—that is, consumer culture—that they
share with postural yoga than from what they claim are static religious
boundaries between themselves and postural yogis, thus negating the
perceived incompatibilities that arise when yoga is constructed for popular consumption.

Yogaphobia

I first used the term *yogaphobia* in a short article responding to what were recent developments in the protests against popularized yoga (see Jain 2010a). Having realized the similarities between certain Christians' fear-inciting and suspicious attitudes toward the popularization of yoga and those who express *Islamophobia*, I turned to Peter Gottschalk and Gabriel Greenberg's definition of Islamophobia for help in operationalizing yogaphobia (Gottschalk and Greenberg 2007: 5).[9] I constructed the following definition:

> *Yogaphobia* is a social anxiety, characterized by suspicion and fear, of modern yoga. It is expressed by certain religious institutions and individuals, emphasizes the incompatibility between yoga and certain doctrines or moral codes, results from and perpetuates essentialist interpretations and Orientalist stereotypes, which are often buttressed by social and political ideologies and agendas, and relies on a sense of otherness, despite many shared cultural qualities.

As early as the nineteenth century, many Christian leaders warned that yoga was not simply about strengthening one's own religious identity and commitments, nor was it simply about attaining physical fitness and reducing stress.[10] Rather, it was a Hindu religious movement that was antithetical to Christianity. Although such Christians have expressed disparate views on yoga's exact nature, they share a polemical stance toward yoga and agree that to some extent Christians who practice yoga endanger their own Christian identities and commitments.

Consider the tragic case involving Ida C. Craddock, introduced in Chapter Two. Craddock was an American social radical and early modern yogi in a period characterized by attempts to legally enforce narrow interpretations of what it meant to be a "Christian nation." Most notable were the attempts of U.S. Postal Inspector Anthony Comstock, who founded the New York Society for the Suppression of Vice and used his position in the postal service to censor whatever he deemed a threat to the Christian morals he identified as American. When Craddock's teachings on yoga conflicted with Comstock's ideals, he sought to enforce laws that would qualify them as illegal. In 1902, after being convicted on charges of obscenity, Craddock spent three torturous months in prison and, with the threat of more prison time, eventually killed herself.

Pierre Bernard, also introduced in Chapter Two, was another turn-of-the-century American social radical, early modern yogi, and victim of yogaphobia. Repeatedly, law enforcement, the media, and the Christian clergy pressured Bernard and his students to forfeit yoga. For years, they were run out of city after city as far as London. Finally, in 1918, Bernard and his students settled in Nyack, New York, where they built an esoteric community housed in the Clarkstown Country Club. Although the Club survived for years, there was a constant stream of yogaphobic responses to what were perceived as exotic and amoral activities at the Club.

Interestingly, Bernard posthumously remains today a victim of yoga-phobia. One evangelical Christian minister and ghost-hunter who goes by the name of Pastor Swope demonizes Bernard in a public blog, *The Paranormal Pastor* (Swope 2008). Swope discusses his days as a student at Nyack College, located on the grounds of what was formerly the Club, and describes the alleged incidents when students, faculty, and staff witnessed paranormal phenomena on campus (Swope 2008).[11] He describes Bernard as a "sex magician" and suspiciously asks, "Did Pierre Bernard unleash something dark that will not die at the Clarkstown Country Club by strange rites and rituals? Or are the ghosts of the Tantric former occupants at odds with the conservative Christian residents who now populate the buildings?" (Swope 2008).

One might expect that yogaphobia would largely disappear after the popularization of postural yoga in the 1960s and that Pastor Swope is merely an outlier, but that is not the case. Marilyn Englund, a yoga instructor, describes how residents responded when she began offering postural yoga classes near Dallas, Texas, in 1979:

> When I first moved to Texas from Chicago in 1979, I was going to set the world on fire by introducing yoga. I immediately took out a classified in *Dallas* magazine for private yoga instruction and massage. That was a big mistake. It brought a lot of phone calls from people who weren't serious. Yoga was something antireligion [sic] to this Bible Belt area, something that people feared would corrupt rather than help. (Leviton 1990: 65)

That incident is in stark contrast to popular attitudes toward yoga today in Dallas and other urban areas (Fig. 6.1). Consider the widely popular *D Magazine* (referred to as Dallas magazine above), which currently features

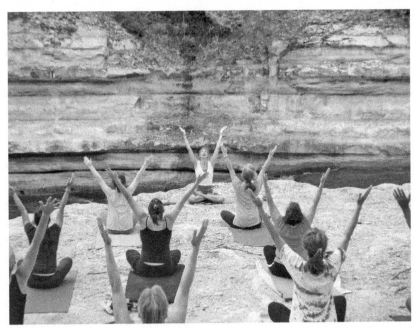

FIGURE 6.1 Yoga 4 Love Community Outdoor Yoga class for Freedom and Gratitude on Independence Day 2010 in Dallas, Texas. Photographed by Lisa Ware and Richard Ware. Released into the public domain. Accessed through Wikimedia Commons.

"Best Yoga" alongside "Best Burger," "Best Brunch," and "Best Hair Salon" in its famous "The Best of Big D" series (*D Magazine* 2011).

Despite such developments, many prominent contemporary Christian institutions and leaders incite fear and suspicion of postural yoga.[12] One example is the Roman Catholic Church, which warned against the "dangers and errors" of fusing Christian and non-Christian meditative methods in 1989 (Congregation for the Doctrine of the Faith 1989: 5). That year the Congregation for the Doctrine of the Faith (CDF), which oversees Church doctrine, sparked controversy when it submitted the "Letter to the Bishops of the Catholic Church on Some Aspects of Christian Meditation" (CDF 1989). The letter was written by Cardinal Joseph Ratzinger (b. 1927; served as Pope Benedict XVI from 2005 to 2013 and currently serves as Pope Emeritus) and was approved for publication by Pope John Paul II (1920–2005).

To be clear, the letter does not discourage Catholics from participating in Eastern methods entirely. In fact, it suggests that methods should not be rejected "simply because they are not Christian," but that they must be compatible with "the Christian conception of prayer" (CDF 1989: 6). Thus it discourages simplistic appropriation but allows for appropriation when Eastern methods are reconstructed "anew" in the Christian context (CDF 1989: 6).

What this means is that the CDF is concerned about the cultivation of experiences that are incompatible with Catholic doctrine. Specifically, the letter warns against adopting a "negative theology" that maintains a notion of an absolute or God without personal qualities (CDF 1989: 5). Catholic Christians should not forget the qualities and deeds through which they can come to know God personally (CDF 1989: 2).

Understandably, the CDF seeks to prevent Catholics from undermining Church doctrine. Yet the letter becomes increasingly fear-inciting when it addresses those Eastern methods that deal with body practices, which are deemed incompatible with Catholic doctrine as well as a threat to basic human stability. Although yoga is not named explicitly, it is implicit that yoga is the object under scrutiny, since it is the preeminent body-centered Eastern method with which contemporary Christians experiment.

The CDF's letter states that those engaged in body practices for the sake of anything beyond mundane physical exercise or relaxation are involved in self-destructive activity. It warns that, unless the practitioner is an advanced mystical and moral adept, no bodily experiences can be legitimately identified as spiritual and points out that Christian writers who have acknowledged the importance of body practices for meditation "avoid the exaggerations and partiality of [Eastern methods], which, however, are often recommended to people today who are not sufficiently prepared" (CDF 1989: 9). It adds that, although some forms of Christian meditation use "psychophysical symbolism," ranging from bodily postures to breathing, such symbolism can become an "idol and thus an obstacle" to experiencing God (CDF 1989: 10). The letter then adopts a polemical tone and becomes even more fear-inciting when it states that body practices "can degenerate into a cult of the body" with severe consequences, including "mental schizophrenia," "psychic disturbance," or "moral deviations" (CDF 1989).

Although the CDF's letter is tinged with yogaphobic discourse, one outspoken Italian Catholic priest, Gabriele Amorth, who was appointed the chief exorcist for the Diocese of Rome in 1986 and founded the International Association of Exorcists in 1990, took yogaphobia farther when in 2011 he warned, "Practicing yoga is Satanic, it leads to evil…" (Squires 2011).

In addition to Catholic cases of yogaphobia, some contemporary, Protestant evangelicals have issued more vocal and sustained attacks on yoga. Their protests range from identifying yoga as self-destructive activity to associating it with Satan. In a 2001 *Today's Christian Woman* article, Jan Brown warns, "Yoga and New Age teach the same lie Satan tempted Eve with in the Garden of Eden: 'You will be as God' (Gen. 3:5), which was designed to keep her (and us) away from the one true God (John 17:3)" (Brown, Jan 2001).[13] Other articles describe individuals who were drawn away from God by yoga. Holly Vicente Robaina recounts Laurette Willis' cautionary tale of how yoga led her into a life of errant New Age practices, loneliness, alcoholism, and promiscuity (Robaina 2005: 40). After years of pain, she became a Christian, burned her New Age books, and gave up yoga. Since 2001, Willis, a public speaker and fitness trainer, has warned Christians about the peril of yoga while promoting a "Christian alternative," which she calls PraiseMoves (PraiseMoves 2010). In a follow-up article, Robaina tells her own story of being seduced by yoga, along with other destructive New Age practices, and the years it took for her to give them up for Christianity (Robaina 2007).[14]

In addition to the yogaphobic maelstrom in widely distributed evangelical publications, some of evangelical Christianity's most influential pastors and scholars have provided fierce yogaphobic responses to Christians practicing yoga. And their yogaphobia can be located within a broader phenomenon, *Hinduphobia*.

Pat Robertson, the notorious television evangelist and founder of the Christian Coalition of America, expressed Hinduphobia in his book *The End of the Age* (1995), an apocalyptic novel in which a devotee of the Hindu god Shiva joins forces with the Antichrist to murder the President of the United States (Robertson 1995).[15] In 2007, Robertson homed in on yoga, describing some aspects as "really spooky" (Robertson 2007).

That same year, in an interview on CNN, John MacArthur, pastor of the Grace Community megachurch in Sun Valley, California, warned Christians against doing yoga, referring to it as a "false religion" (MacArthur 2007). Then in 2010, Mark Driscoll, pastor of the Mars Hill megachurch in Seattle, Washington, told the following to a live audience:

Yoga is demonic…It's absolute paganism…Yoga and meditation and Easternism is [sic] all opening to demonism…if you just sign up for a little yoga class, you're signing up for a little demon class.

That's what you're doing. And Satan doesn't care if you stretch as long as you go to hell. (Driscoll 2010)

One of the most controversial cases of yogaphobia, and perhaps the one having the greatest direct consequences for Americans actually doing yoga, involves the Encinitas, California, public schools. In 2013, some parents in Encinitas began a campaign to remove recently introduced postural yoga classes from their public schools, arguing that yoga promotes Hinduism. The parents worked in conjunction with the National Center for Law & Policy (NCLP), an evangelical Christian civil liberties organization. The NCLP sued the Encinitas Union School District (EUSD) for introducing religion into the curriculum in order to promote a certain religion—that is, Hinduism.

The NCLP targets the Jois Foundation, a nonprofit organization founded in memory of Krishna Pattabhi Jois, the person responsible for popularizing Ashtanga yoga. The Jois Foundation gave the EUSD a $533,000 grant to support postural yoga classes for students. Resources for yoga at the school also included financial support from the University of Virginia and the University of San Diego, where scholars have studied the effects of yoga on children's health. The NCLP responded with criticism, suggesting the Jois Foundation is a Hindu institution.

In her expert witness brief, religious studies scholar Candy Gunther Brown provided support for the NCLP's argument, suggesting, "The practices taught by the EUSD yoga curriculum promote and advance religion, including Hinduism—whether or not these practices are taught using religious or Hindu language" (Brown, Candy Gunther 2013: 4). In response, representatives from the school district insisted that the curriculum is designed in such a way as to exclude any Hindu religious elements. Timothy Baird, the EUSD Superintendent, argued, "To be unconstitutional, we would have to be promoting religion and religious instruction in our program. That just isn't happening. What we are promoting is physical activity and overall wellness" (Holpuch 2013).

These pastors and organizations do not exhaust the Christian opposition to yoga. In a conversation with Albert Mohler, President of the Southern Baptist Theological Seminary, about the popularization of yoga, Douglas Groothuis, Professor of Philosophy at Denver Seminary, suggested that the "alien spiritual practice" of yoga cannot "be incorporated into a faithful, biblical way of life" (Groothuis 2010). He argued that the "point of yoga" is to transform consciousness in order to realize union with the underlying essence of all things according to Hindu non-dualist thought, which makes yoga incompatible with Christian theology (Groothuis 2010). Groothuis suggested "the [school of yoga] that has the biggest impact on the west" is nondualist. In defense of that vision, he quoted Swami Vivekananda, introduced in Chapter Two.[16] Vivekananda was a nineteenth-century Hindu reformer, missionary to the United States, and Indian nationalist who promoted a form of yoga based on a modern interpretation of advaita vedanta (a Hindu nondualist philosophical school). According to Groothuis, Vivekananda's argument that "the highest meditation is to think of nothing" suggests that yoga is in conflict with Christianity, which calls on us to "meditate on the truths that God has revealed" and "to grow in our knowledge of God...through the life, death [*sic*] resurrection of Jesus Christ" (Groothuis 2010).

Groothuis resorted to polemical discourse in further generalizations about postural yogis. He argued that "the yoga people," though they may first become interested in yoga for physical and psychological benefits, are in fact looking for "the telos that is the essential purpose of yoga" within themselves (Groothuis 2010). He added, "yoga aims at the elimination of the body, it is a depersonalizing, deindividualizing, dehumanizing practice" (Groothuis 2010).

Mohler became the dominant contemporary yogaphobic voice when his September 20, 2010, blog post, in which he warned Christians not to choose yoga, made headlines (Mohler 2010c). Like the other Christians discussed above, Mohler insists that yoga cannot be separated from Hinduism, a conflation that functions as the main premise for both dimensions of his Christian yogaphobic position: the doctrinal argument (that yoga is at odds with Christian doctrine) and the nationalist argument (that yoga undermines the Christian essence of American culture).

Mohler writes:

> When Christians practice yoga, they must either deny the reality of what yoga represents or fail to see the contradictions between their Christian commitments and their embrace of yoga. The contradictions are not few, nor are they peripheral. (Mohler 2010c)

Mohler is disturbed by what he perceives as the yoga doctrine that the body is a means to experience the divine. Such a doctrine conflicts with his idea that Christians should rely only on biblical scripture as a means to understanding God (Mohler 2010b; Mohler 2010c). More specifically, he suggests that yoga requires one to overcome the body as a way to salvation and that this is "just not Christianity" (Mohler 2010b).

In addition to being disturbed by Christians adopting what he perceives as yoga's singular approach to the body, Mohler disapproves of yoga's meditative components. Like the CDF, Mohler suggests that the meditative components of "Eastern religions" are about emptying the mind. Whereas the CDF argues that Christians should meditate on the qualities of God, Mohler insists that Christians should meditate on scripture (Mohler 2008).

Mohler, however, goes beyond an argument for doctrinal incompatibility and turns to explicit suspicion- and fear-inciting discourse. Yoga is a "rejection" and "reversal" of the Gospel (Mohler 2010b). In other words, yoga is not just incompatible with Christianity but threatens Christianity. To demonstrate how yoga functions as a distraction from true religion, he asks, "What in the world does yoga promise after death?" (Mohler 2010b). Mohler's response is "absolute non-consciousness" (Mohler 2010b). Because it distracts from true religion, which provides better answers to such questions, yoga is dangerous.

Mohler suggests that any non-Christian form of meditation is a "dangerous distraction" and an "empty promise" and is essentially selfish (Mohler 2008). He argues that yoga is characterized by "theological confusion," "spiritual smattering," and "fadicism" and that whether or not Christians practice yoga has nothing to do with medical benefits or its complex history but with whether or not they have come to know Christ (Mohler 2010b).

Mohler compares Christian postural yogis to Gnostic Christians, and, like many early Christians who opposed the Gnostics, he resorts to polemics, arguing:

> [The American cult of health] is a concentration upon the self that is not spiritually healthy and yoga for many people I think becomes the entry drug recognized or not into more troubling forms of spirituality and spiritual confusion. (Mohler 2010b)

In another article, he discusses a study showing that New Age religion is growing in Britain (Mohler 2004).[17] His concern is with New Age religion generally, but he includes yoga in that category. Mohler cites the study as proof that New Age religion threatens Christianity and thus should serve as a "wake up call to the Christian Church" (Mohler 2004). He ends by warning Americans, "Don't think it can't happen here" (Mohler 2004).

Mohler's position demonstrates how yogaphobia incites suspicion and fear for the advancement of social and political agendas. He considers the popularization of yoga to be a symptom of the "post-modern confusion of America" (Mohler 2010b). The fact that, in two separate discussions on yoga, Mohler brings up First Lady Michelle Obama's choice to add yoga to the events at the annual White House Easter Egg Roll (associating the Obama administration with the post-Christian nation he so fears) confirms that Mohler's yogaphobia is one symptom of a broader movement to construct the United States according to a narrow vision of what it means to be a "Christian nation" (Mohler 2010b; Mohler 2010c). Many of the contemporary players in that movement participate in the Islamophobic smears that Barack Obama is secretly Muslim and even anti-Christian.[18] The popularization of yoga is perceived as a symptom that the Christian nation is in decline. In Mohler's words:

> The story of yoga [in America] is a twisted tale of how something that is so essentially rooted in Hinduism could become part of American popular culture and increasingly a part of the lives of many who would identify themselves as Christians—it's a large number of persons. (Mohler 2010b)

The story of yoga in the United States is a "twisted tale" from Mohler's perspective because he defines American culture as essentially Christian and yoga as essentially Hindu. But the popularization of yoga, according to Mohler, is just one symptom of how Hinduism threatens American culture. Enter Hinduphobia once again. Part of the problem with yoga is that it comes from India. In discussing yoga's Indian roots, Mohler characterizes it as "almost manically syncretistic" (Mohler 2010c). He warns that if that syncretism is allowed to further infect the United States, the result will be the unthinkable: a "post-Christian" nation (Mohler 2010c). He is disturbed by the fact that, according to a 2008 Pew Forum survey, Americans are becoming increasingly open to the idea that "many religions can lead to eternal life" (Mohler 2009; for the survey, see *The Pew Forum* 2008). Associating this position with Hinduism, which he considers radically relativistic and in conflict with Christian exclusivism, he warns that the United States is becoming a "nation of Hindus" (Mohler 2009).

According to Mohler, the increasing Hinduization of the United States could be "nothing less than catastrophic" (Mohler 2009). Ultimately, he argues, if the Church does not "regain its theological sanity and evangelistic courage to resist this trend," then "being described as a nation of Hindus will be the least of our problems" (Mohler 2009). He thus conflates Church agenda with national agenda in response to social trends, and the perceived incursion of Hinduism—especially in the form of yoga—is a trend of ultimate concern.

Hindu Origins

When a *New York Times* front-page article brought to mainstream attention a Hindu organization's campaign to raise awareness of yoga's so-called Hindu origins (Vitello 2010), Mohler interpreted it as a "vindication" for his own position on yoga (Mohler 2010a). The Hindu American Foundation (HAF), a Minneapolis-based organization that advocates for Hindus living in the United States, introduced the "Take Back Yoga— Bringing to Light Yoga's Hindu Roots" campaign in January 2010. Because an argument for the Hindu origins of yoga is foundational to the HAF's position, I call it the *Hindu origins position*. It utilizes polemical discourse, which in its most extreme forms includes accusations that the popularization of yoga amounts to the "rape" and "theft" of yoga (A. Shukla 2010c; A. Shukla and Shah 2011).

It is not surprising that Mohler perceived a vindication in the Hindu origins position; after all, it shares key qualities with Mohler's Christian yogaphobic position. Both reify homogenous definitions of yoga as Hindu and protest against the popularization of postural yoga, which is perceived to dramatically ignore or dilute yoga's Hindu essence.

The two positions also differ in important ways. On the one hand, Christian protesters cast doubt on postural yoga's potential merits and attack what is perceived as a homogenous yoga system. On the other hand, advocates of the Hindu origins position valorize what they perceive as a homogenous yoga system by reifying its associations with what they deem authentic Hinduism and denouncing those forms—especially those of postural yoga—that deviate. Rather than being concerned with discouraging non-Hindus from practicing yoga, Hindu protesters primarily have two different concerns. First, they are concerned that popularized systems of postural yoga are corruptions of what they consider authentic yoga. And second, they are concerned that Hinduism does not get due credit when postural yogis coopt yoga.

In the same way that the history of modern yoga features earlier cases of Christian yogaphobia, it also features earlier cases of the Hindu origins position. Certain nineteenth- and early-twentieth-century Hindu reformers and nationalists targeted certain yoga practitioners for what they thought was yoga done wrong. They prescribed an alternative that they valorized as a rational, philosophical system. In Chapter Two, we discussed those who expressed contempt for certain types of yoga based on a bifurcation between yoga's philosophical and meditative techniques, often equated with classical yoga or raja yoga, and its physical techniques, often equated with hatha yoga. They dismissed hatha yoga as inauthentic for what were considered extreme, ascetic body-centered practices.

Most significantly for the history of modern yoga, Vivekananda constructed and disseminated a system of modern yoga, which he called raja yoga, in response to dominant Euro-American and Christian modes of thought. He participated in Hindu reform efforts to familiarize Indian, American, and European elites with an image of yoga distinct from hatha yoga.[19] His raja yoga was the antithesis of the body-centered practices that many associated with yoga. Although he did appropriate some physical components, he did so only with regard to belief in the existence of a subtle body (de Michelis 2004: 166–167). In this way, he argued, the yogic manipulation of subtle energy could function as a healing agent (de Michelis 2004: 163–168). Physical benefits, however, were inferior to what he considered the true aim of yoga: spiritual development (Vivekananda 1992 [1896]: 20).

Vivekananda at times even used the Christian Bible as a tool for demonizing body-centered yoga practices (Singleton 2010: 74–75). In one instance, he cited the Sermon on the Mount in the Gospel of Matthew when Jesus tells his audience to set their mind on God's kingdom and not on the future (Matthew 6:33–34) to support his argument that any yoga tradition concerned with enhancing the body for health or longevity was not authentic (Singleton 2010: 74–75).

Vivekananda's interpretation of advaita vedanta functioned as the so-called rational foundation of yoga. He maintained that any version of yoga other than the rationalist one he prescribed was a corruption of its true form, arguing "the more modern the commentator, the greater the mistakes he makes, while the more ancient the writer, the more rational he is" (Vivekananda 1992 [1896]: 20).

Vivekananda's revisionist historical narrative about yoga thrived until the second half of the twentieth century, when body-centered postural yoga became increasingly popular.[20] But even advocates of postural yoga appealed to Hindu origins. The body-centered practices equated with hatha yoga were now reconstructed and medicalized in ways that made them modern fitness techniques deemed original to Hinduism (Alter 2004; Singleton 2010). Hindu nationalists assimilated Euro-American physical culture and associated it with yoga (Singleton 2010). In this way, they valorized postural yoga by prescribing it as an indigenous form of physical fitness.

Today, the Hindu origins position is largely based on sound objections to popular stereotypes. Protestors are concerned that stereotypes prevent postural yogis from acknowledging yoga's Hindu origins, which in turn serves to disenfranchise Hindus from their tradition (A. Shukla 2010c). Aseem Shukla, co-founder and board member of the HAF and one of the loudest voices for the Take Back Yoga campaign, argues that Hinduism is popularly identified with "holy cows," "warring gods," and "wandering ascetics" (A. Shukla 2010c). And an official statement by the HAF refers to a popular caricature of Hinduism as nothing but "caste, cows and curry" (HAF 2009b). As articulated by Suhag Shukla, the popular *Yoga Journal* and much of the yoga industry generally avoid the "unmarketable 'H-word'" (S. Shukla 2011). Many argue that, because of stereotypes about Hinduism, postural yogis talk about yoga as "ancient Indian," "Eastern," or "Sanskritic" rather than as Hindu (A. Shukla 2010c; S. Shukla 2011).

Although such stereotypes are unquestionably problematic, advocates of the Hindu origins position offer just one more inaccurate, homogenizing vision of Hinduism. Mirroring Orientalist condemnations of Hindu body practices and rituals, they construct a reified Hinduism in line with other conceptions of "neo-Hinduism," which promote what is valorized as "true" Hindu spirituality as opposed to irrational corruptions. For example, Shukla argues that stereotypes about Hinduism should be replaced with the following qualities he deems truly representative of Hinduism: "arduous" yoga postures, "the unity of divinity," and Patanjali, author of the *Yoga Sutras*, which provides the "philosophical basis of Yoga practice today" (A. Shukla 2010c).

Although advocates of the Hindu origins position are concerned with the lack of references to Hinduism in popular yoga contexts, their campaign targets specific popular brands, styles, and teachers, such as Transcendental Meditation, *Yoga Journal*, Deepak Chopra, and Bikram Yoga, that they believe are paragons of this marketing strategy (A. Shukla 2010c; A. Shukla and Shah 2011). Consider Deepak Chopra's triumph in the market for South Asian cultural wares. Chopra's success in marketing yoga as "spiritual" but not "religious" or "Hindu" has been phenomenal. Consequently, he is a common target of advocates for the Hindu origins position, who contrast figures like Chopra with Vivekananda, whose agenda they perceive as compatible with their own (for Chopra's response, see Chopra 2010a; Chopra 2010b).

Protestors are particularly bothered by the argument that yoga is not Hindu because it is "spiritual, not religious," suggesting that it buttresses profit-driven marketing campaigns. Shukla and Shah argue that marketers emphasize yoga's benefits for mental and physical health without mention of "that pariah term: 'Hinduism'" (A. Shukla and Shah 2011). Ramesh Rao adds that "savvy marketers" avoid the term *Hinduism* in order to appease Christians who want to practice yoga and simultaneously "hang on to Jesus" (Rao 2010).

Some go so far as to argue that yoga is the "intellectual property" of Hinduism, and thus the yoga market amounts to the "theft of yoga" (A. Shukla 2010c). Shukla adds:

> [Yoga is] a victim of overt intellectual property theft, absence of trademark protections and the facile complicity of generations of Hindu yogis, gurus, swamis and others that offered up a religion's spiritual wealth at the altar of crass commercialism. (A. Shukla 2010c)

Even the Indian government joined the ownership debate. The government-run Traditional Knowledge Digital Library (TKDL) created a database of thirteen hundred yoga postures believed to be documented in ancient Indian texts (Sinha 2011). The TKDL's hope is that the database will function as a reference point for patent offices all over the world to check each time someone applies for a patent on a particular yoga posture or sequence. The aim is to prevent yoga marketers from claiming ownership and consequently profiting off something that is believed to have ancient Indian origins. The TKDL is especially concerned about Bikram Choudhury's patent on the twenty-six posture sequence of his Bikram Yoga (see Fish 2006; Srinivas 2007).[21] According to the creator of the TKDL, V. P. Gupta, all of Bikram Yoga's postures were mentioned in ancient Indian texts (Fish 2006; Srinivas 2007).[22]

Although some voices of the Hindu origins position argue in terms of Hindu *ownership*, most voices prefer to argue in terms of Hindu *origins*. According to this position, neither Hinduism nor India owns yoga (HAF 2009a; Shah 2010; S. Shukla 2011). Nevertheless yoga is originally Hindu (Shah 2010; S. Shukla 2010; S. Shukla 2011). Suhag Shukla explains:

> ...in practicing the universally applicable core concepts of Hinduism, codeword "yoga", a Christian can come closer to Christ; a Jew closer to Yahweh; a Muslim closer to Allah; and last but not least, a Hindu closer to Krishna (or Shiva or Shakti or Brahman, or whatever name the Wise may call It). (S. Shukla 2010)

In short, yoga is Hindu but is beneficial for members of all religions. Conflating yoga with the "core concepts of Hinduism," they maintain that yoga dates back over five thousand years to the Indus Valley Civilization, that the religion of that civilization was an early form of Hinduism, and that yoga's origins can thus be traced back to Hinduism, from which it is forever inseparable (HAF 2009b).[23] They cite narrowly selected texts, including the *Yoga Sutras*, the *Bhagavad Gita*, and the *Hatha Yoga Pradipika* in addition to texts by the contemporary yoga guru, B. K. S. Iyengar, and point out what they consider the Hindu theological dimensions of these texts, concluding that yoga is always a Hindu "means of spiritual attainment" (HAF 2009b). Shukla and Shah concisely articulate the argument for the perceived inseparable Hindu–experiential dimension of yoga: "Yoga, in its path of regaining mastery over the body, mind and intellect, does not offer ways to believe in God; it offer [sic] ways to know God" (A. Shukla and Shah 2011).

So yoga provides Hindu "ways to know God" and yet, according to the Hindu origins position, Hinduism receives neither recognition nor appreciation for contributing yoga to the world. And opponents of postural yoga warn that it gets worse: Postural yogis corrupt yoga. In a polemical attack on American postural yogis, Shukla and Shah argue, "For these self-indulgent appropriators of Yoga in the US, the end-all-and-be-all of Yoga is *asana*-based classes" (A. Shukla and Shah 2011). Postural yoga is considered illegitimate and prescribed by marketers concerned with profit alone (Shah 2010). The HAF suggests:

Yoga, as an integral part of Hindu philosophy, is not simply physical exercise in the form of various *asanas* and *pranayama*, but is in fact a Hindu way of life. The ubiquitous use of the word "Yoga" to describe what in fact is simply an *asana* exercise is not only misleading, but has led to and is fueling a problematic delinking of Yoga and Hinduism...(HAF 2009b)

Echoing Vivekananda, representatives of the HAF argue that authentic yoga is raja yoga as found in Patanjali's *Yoga Sutras* with its eight limbs, of which posture is only one (HAF 2009b; A. Shukla 2010c). They equate postural yoga with hatha yoga, which they, like Vivekananda, denounce for focusing exclusively on body-centered practices and ignoring moral and spiritual dimensions (HAF 2009b; A. Shukla 2010c).

The HAF's campaign prescribes yoga not only for health, but also, and more importantly, as a Hindu practice. Thus it approves of yoga as a means to health, "But the Foundation argues that the full potential of the physiological, intellectual and spiritual benefits of *asana* would be increased manifold if practiced as a component of the holistic practice of Yoga" (HAF 2009b). In other words, all yogis should practice all eight limbs as prescribed by Patanjali according to their selective reading of the *Yoga Sutras*.

Like the Christian yogaphobic position, the Hindu origins position goes hand in hand with a polemical attack on the New Age movement. Advocates of the Hindu origins position describe popularized forms of yoga as steeped in "new age blather" and the "intellectual gobbledygook of New Age platitudes" (A. Shukla 2010b; A. Shukla and Shah 2011).

According to protestors, Hinduism and authentic yoga are synonymous. But anyone can practice yoga as long as he or she does so with caution:

But be forewarned. Yogis say that the dedicated practice of yoga will subdue the restless mind, lessen one's cravings for the mundane material world and put one on the path of self-realization—that each individual is a spark of the Divine. Expect conflicts if you are sold on the exclusivist claims of Abrahamic faiths—that their God awaits the arrival of only His chosen few at heaven's gate—since yoga shows its own path to spiritual enlightenment to all seekers regardless of affiliation. (A. Shukla 2010c)

Given such fear-inciting warnings about the narrowly conceived Hindu essence of yoga and the inevitable Hinduization of any yogi, it is no wonder Mohler finds bedfellows in advocates of the Hindu origins position.

Essentialist Discourse and Strategies

As I peruse the many protests against the popularization of yoga, I see a series of streams crossing, and, if one evaluates any one of those streams without considering it in the context of a larger movement, then it may come across as an outlying voice. Furthermore, Christian and Hindu protesters have a variety of home organizations and leaders that they affiliate with or follow closely, the missions of which are different.[24] Yet protestors participate in a shared broad-based movement that is conditioned by certain assumptions. When considered together, therefore, it becomes apparent that these voices share a discourse and strategies toward a common goal: defining postural yoga in terms of a Hindu essence as a protest against its popularization. Their discourse and strategies are in conflict with historical experience, which Said convincingly argues suggests that "all cultures are involved in one another; none is single and pure, all are hybrid, heterogeneous, extraordinarily differentiated, and unmonolithic" (Said 1994: xxv).[25]

One way to understand the striking intersections between the Christian yogaphobic position and the Hindu origins position is by evaluating the strategies they share with the nineteenth-century movement responsible for defining *Hinduism*. Attempts to define Hinduism began with European Orientalists (Inden 1992; Smith, David 2003), but the specifics of what that notion looked like resulted from a discourse between Orientalists and elite Hindu reformers (Halbfass 1988; Lopez 1995; King 1999; Viswanathan 2003; Pennington 2005).[26] With regard to nineteenth-century Indian intellectuals, Wilhelm Halbfass argues:

> The Indians reinterpreted key concepts of their traditional self-understanding, adjusting them to Western modes of understanding. By appealing to the West, by using its conceptual tools, they tried to secure and defend the identity and continuity of their tradition. (Halbfass 1988: 173)

According to Richard King, such conceptions have allowed "Hindus to turn Western colonial discourses to their own advantage" (King 1999: 142).

The result, according to King, was a definition of Hinduism "in terms of a normative paradigm of religion" based on a bifurcation between the so-called superior qualities that Orientalists attributed to religions of "the West" and the so-called inferior qualities that they attributed to religions of "the East" (King 1999: 101).[27]

In response to Orientalist critiques of "the East," certain Hindu reformers postulated "an ahistorical 'essence'" to Hinduism characterized by many of the qualities that Orientalists attributed to "the West" (King 1999: 104).[28] Having eliminated many traditions and qualities of Indian religions, they conflated a sanitized vision of Hinduism with the rational religion they found in their selective readings of texts like the *Upanishads*, the *Yoga Sutras*, and the *Bhagavad Gita*.[29] Such texts received new primacy in what was perceived as a Hindu canon, which was read through a narrow, modern interpretation of advaita vedanta (King 1999: 102–105). Whatever did not fit into their notion of authentic Hinduism was relegated to a form of Hinduism considered "a corrupt shadow of its former self" (King 1999: 105).

This systematic censorship continues among some scholars of Indian religions today, as evidenced by responses to scholarship by religious studies scholars, such as Hugh B. Urban and Jeffrey J. Kripal. Urban and Kripal have both convincingly argued that Vivekananda rewrote the life of his guru, Ramakrishna, to make Ramakrishna fit into his narrow, homogenous vision of authentic Hinduism. He did this primarily by denying Ramakrishna's involvement in tantra and hatha yoga (Kripal 1998; Urban 2003: 161–163). Kripal and Urban, in addition to other contemporary religious studies scholars, including Wendy Doniger, Paul B. Courtright, and David Gordon White, whose attention to aspects of Hindu traditions that were not conducive to the homogenous vision elite Hindu intellectuals sought to perpetuate, have been subject to repeated incendiary attacks.[30] The debate has culminated in nationalist pleas for Indians to take control over how the story of Indian history is told. Dilip K. Chakrabarti, for example, made such a plea, citing William Dalrymple: "One should protect one's own history and fight for it by tooth and claw, as others will always try to change it" (Chakrabarti 2009, cited by Samuel 2011: 349). Geoffrey Samuel provides a constructive response to such pleas:

...there is a natural tendency for those of us who have been engaged in the literature on postcolonial thought to sympathize with such attempts to repatriate Indian history. However, ultimately the history of Indic religions is not just the property of the modern Indian state or of the people who currently live there, and it would be to everyone's disadvantage were it to be subsumed into a particular nationalist project. (Samuel 2011: 349)

Just as the notion of a homogenous Hinduism resulted from discourse between Orientalists and elite Hindu reformers, so the contemporary construction of a homogenous yoga tradition results from a discourse between the Christian yogaphobic position and the Hindu origins position. And, in a way similar to how Orientalist and reformist attempts to define Hinduism revealed more about those movements' subjectivity than about any reality underlying representations of Hinduism, the discourse through which the Hindu origins position and the Christian yogaphobic position define yoga reveals more about protesters' subjectivity than about any reality underlying their representations of yoga.

Protesters essentialize yoga's religious identity as Hindu. For example, Shukla warns that Christian postural yogis should "expect conflicts" since yoga amounts to a Hindu path to enlightenment (A. Shukla 2010c), and Groothuis warns that Christian postural yogis will inevitably end up pursuing an experience of Brahman (Groothuis 2010). Yet, as noted in Chapter One, for at least two thousand years in South Asia, people from various ideological and practical religious cultures "reinvented" yoga in their own images (White 2012: 2).[31] Furthermore, the interreligious and intercultural exchanges—primarily among Hindu, Buddhist, and Jain traditions—throughout the history of yoga in South Asia problematize the identification of yoga as Hindu.[32]

Having assumed the Hindu identity of yoga, protesters essentialize the aim of yoga when, for example, Mohler reduces it to "absolute non-consciousness," Shukla and Shah reduce it to "[knowing] God" (A. Shukla and Shah 2011), or Groothuis insists:

[T]he essential point, the goal of yoga is not the purification of the body or the beautification of the physique, [but] a change in consciousness... wherein one finds oneself at one with the ultimate reality which in Hinduism is Brahman (Groothuis 2010).[33]

Although South Asian premodern yoga systems are often soteriologies that aim toward release from suffering existence, and they require the practitioner to manipulate the mind–body complex, the details regarding how the aim and requirements are conceptualized and the methods for attaining them vary dramatically.[34]

The history of postural yoga also problematizes the identification of yoga as Hindu. As discussed in preceding chapters, that history is a paragon of cultures being "involved in one another" in the process of constructing something new in response to transnational ideas and movements. In the first half of the twentieth century, postural yoga emerged "as a hybridized product of colonial India's dialogical encounter with the worldwide physical culture movement" (Singleton 2010: 80). In fact, postural yoga was the "cultural successor" of "established methods of stretching and relaxing" that were already common in parts of Western Europe and the United States (Singleton 2010: 154). Postural yoga is a twentieth-century product, the aims of which include modern conceptions of physical fitness, stress reduction, beauty, and overall well-being (Alter 2004; de Michelis 2004; Strauss 2005; Newcombe 2007; Singleton 2010).[35] For these reasons, Geoffrey Samuel argues, "[Modern yoga] should be judged in its own terms, not in terms of its closeness to some presumably more authentic Indian practice...the process both at the Indian and at the western ends was and is one of creative adaptation rather than of literal transmission" (Samuel 2007: 178).

In addition to understanding the intersections between the Christian yogaphobic position and the Hindu origins position in terms of their revisionist historical accounts, one can understand them in terms of the extent to which they serve the exclusivist and evaluative judgments of religious fundamentalism. They are exempla of how different forms of religious fundamentalism, or in Said's term, *religious enthusiasm*, "belong essentially to the same world, feed off one another, emulate and war against one another schizophrenically, and—most seriously—are as ahistorical and as intolerant as one another" (Said 2004: 51).

The memory of Orientalists' and Hindu reformers' exclusivist and evaluative judgments of certain South Asian traditions, including body-centered yoga systems, is embedded in contemporary popular culture, so it is not shocking that postural yoga is subject to similar judgments. Just as early analyses of Hindu mysticism constructed mysticism in a way that made it decontextualized, elitist, antisocial, otherworldly, and domesticated based on a differentiation between the "mystical East" and the "rational West" (King 1999: 24), so protesters differentiate between postural yoga and authentic Christianity or authentic Hinduism.[36] Mohler, on the one hand, contrasts the postural yogi with the authentic

Christian when he essentializes the method and aim of yoga, suggesting that it requires one to overcome the body as a way to salvation, which is "just not Christianity" (Mohler 2010b). When the HAF argues that yoga is "not simply physical exercise" (HAF 2009b), it contrasts the postural yogi with the authentic Hindu.

Protesters freely select from yoga those objects and texts in service to their evaluative agendas. Advocates of the Christian yogaphobic position emphasize references to Hindu deities in the titles of some postures and the use of the body as a means to nondualist mystical experience.[37] By means of this selective strategy, postural yoga is deemed inferior and threatening to Christian doctrine.

In the same way that Orientalists used the notion of the "mystical East" to legitimate colonialism and provoke fear of Indian self-rule, advocates of the Christian yogaphobic position rely on a fear-inciting vision of yoga and identity politics to justify an agenda to prevent social, political, and religious boundary crossing. More specifically, Mohler's vision aims to recreate an historical moment in which a particular version of Christianity functioned as the dominant political and social voice in the United States, and Hindu and New Age traditions were marginalized. His fear of a "post-Christian" nation assumes that the United States has its cultural origins in Christianity, an assumption that is just as historically problematic as arguing that yoga has its origins in Hinduism (on religions in American history, see Albanese 2012).[38]

Advocates of the Hindu origins position also resort to a selective strategy in order to argue that postural yoga is inferior to authentic Hinduism. Protesters argue that postural yogis' focus on physical fitness and their consumer preference-based approach to yoga are incompatible with authentic Hindu yoga, which is philosophical and meditational and aims toward a theistic experience of God.[39] For instance, they point to Patanjali's *Yoga Sutras* as yoga's ur-text. This selective strategy aims to erase the heterogeneity of yoga's history and models the exclusivist strategies of Vivekananda.[40] All of this contributes to a long history of identity politics among Hindu reformers and nationalists concerned with narrowing the definition of who counts as an authentic Hindu.

Definitions of religious phenomena continuously shift according to shifting cultural, political, and discursive contexts. Just as, according to Talal Asad, "there cannot be a universal definition of religion, not only because its constituent elements and relationships are historically specific, but because that definition is itself the historical product of discursive processes" (Asad 1993: 29), so there cannot be a universal definition of yoga. Yet advocates of the Christian yogaphobic position and the Hindu origins position ignore the dynamic history of yoga. They imagine themselves as transhistorical players in homogenous traditions whose boundaries are in need of defense. And the threatening objects they identify are predicated on those objects' conformity to—or, for the Hindu origins position, corruption of—a list of essential qualities that they identify as Hindu, ignoring the insider realities of living practitioners of postural yoga.

Unintentional Truths

The strategies of the Christian yogaphobic position and the Hindu origins position problematically ignore the realities of the idiosyncratic methods and aims of postural yoga as well as its historical development when they deny the intersecting cultural contexts from which it emerged. As I suggested in preceding chapters, the methods and aims of postural yoga dramatically vary. Yet protesters are right that the question of whether or not individuals should choose postural yoga as a part of their physical fitness routines does betray certain truths about our current cultural moment.

For those who protest the popularization of yoga, the question betrays that postural yoga poses a threat to what they perceive as bounded traditions, namely Christianity and Hinduism. I suggest, however, that the protesters unintentionally betray truths about the qualities of the current cultural moment, that is of consumer culture, that they *share* with the very thing they protest against. In other words, in a way similar to how the discourse through which the Hindu origins position and the Christian yogaphobic position define yoga reveals more about the protesters' own fundamentalist and revisionist historical subjectivities than about any reality underlying their representations of yoga, we also learn about protesters' subjectivities as participants in consumer culture. This becomes apparent as we uncover their consumer dialect, which in turn reveals qualities that include self-consciousness regarding the key role of choice in constructing one's self-identity and lifestyle, as well as an approach to the body that deems its enhancement through physical fitness a valuable part of self-development.

As a way of moving beyond the essentialist conceptions of yoga and therefore taking seriously the somatic, semantic, and symbolic fields of meaning that postural yoga generates for millions of contemporary individuals who do yoga, I suggested in preceding chapters that we evaluate postural yoga not in terms of transmission from or mere commodification of earlier yoga systems, but as an often religious product of contemporary culture (that is, consumer culture). It turns out that one of the consequences of adopting that approach is that the boundaries and incompatibilities between contemporary popular forms of postural yoga and the reified categories of Hinduism and Christianity break down, since contemporary Hindu and Christian individuals and movements share the same consumer dialect as is dominant in the postural yoga world. In other words, a pervasive consumer culture is reflected by postural yoga, the Christian yogaphobic position, and the Hindu origins position and, therefore, negates the perceived incompatibilities that arise when yoga is constructed for popular consumption.

In their fear that misguided individuals are increasingly choosing yoga, opponents of postural yoga acknowledge the fact that participants in consumer culture pick and choose from a variety of practices and worldviews, choosing them much like they choose commodities. Consumers choose from a variety of yoga systems, but choice certainly does not stop there. In the area of physical fitness alone, they choose from an endless list of regimens believed to enhance the body in ways that suit individual desires and needs. Just as a single consumer can choose to attend a YMCA spin class, a Bikram Yoga class, a tai chi class, or all of the above, that consumer can also choose to attend Driscoll's Mars Hill Church or a different church or place of worship from a wide variety of possibilities.

Protesters against popularized yoga recognize that choice is a fact of contemporary culture and perceive it as a challenge to boundaries they want to maintain. Thus, it is the fact that choice becomes an imperative in every area of life in consumer culture that stirred both the popularization of yoga (the heterogeneity of products in the market made it possible for a wide variety of individuals to choose it) as well as the protests against it (protesters have reacted against choice because it threatens religious boundaries).

Since protests emerged from the same cultural context that gave birth to the popularization of yoga, it is not surprising that postural yogis and their opponents share a cultural dialect. Specifically, the question they pose, namely whether or not individuals should choose postural yoga as part of their physical fitness regimen, betrays the cultural assumption that individuals should choose a physical fitness regimen at all. In other words, both postural yogis and their opponents assume that *physical fitness is worth choosing.* They all reflect a reality of consumer culture: Physical fitness products are deemed valuable to self-development.

So postural yoga does not reflect the invasion of a foreign product into the lives of Christians, nor does it reflect a merely profit-driven market that corrupts authentic Hinduism. It is, rather, a reflection of dominant trends in consumer culture. Since postural yoga's central feature is an approach to the body that treats its enhancement as part of self-development, an approach to the body that is valorized in consumer culture, it is not a coincidence that it has increasingly attained global popularity since the second half of the twentieth century. As I suggested in preceding chapters, postural yoga is in part a product of consumer culture, hence the absence of anything that looks like it in the history of yoga prior to the twentieth century.

Although contemporary Christian protesters against the popularization of yoga perceive a complete incompatibility between their approaches to the body and that found in postural yoga, none actually exists. Consider how protesters pick and choose what are perceived as the less threatening and even appealing aspects of postural yoga. In this way they assume the value of physical fitness. Mohler himself suggests, "There is nothing wrong with physical exercise, and yoga positions in themselves are not the main issue" (Mohler 2010c), an assertion that is consistent with those of other evangelical opponents of yoga. Robertson encourages Christians to engage in non-yoga stretching (Robertson 2007), and Driscoll follows his statement that yoga is demonic by noting the value of stretching and exercise, things that can even be "biblical" (Driscoll 2010). As discussed in more detail in Chapter Five, some Christian protesters of postural yoga come up with Christian "alternatives," such as Willis' PraiseMoves.

Advocates of the Hindu origins position agree that physical fitness is key to self-development. Their protests do not question postural yogis' valorization of physical fitness but suggest that yoga's physical benefits should be understood as one component of a "Hindu way of life" (HAF 2009b). They are quick to valorize the physical and psychological benefits of postural yoga but are also quick to insist that they are not sufficient:

> Indeed, yogis believe that to focus on the physicality of yoga without the spirituality is utterly rudimentary and deficient. Sure, practicing postures alone with a focus on breathing techniques will quiet the mind, tone the body, and increase flexibility—even help

children with Attention Deficit Disorder—but [it] will miss the mark on holistic healing and wellness. (A. Shukla 2010c)

Protesters' intention is to assert incompatibilities between their world-views and postural yoga and to warn Christians and Hindus that the popularization of yoga threatens religious boundaries. Instead they betray important truths about their own subjectivity as participants in consumer culture, much of which they share with the very cultural product they protest.

Conclusion

Resentment or protest of postural yoga emerges from a distorted view of history that serves a fierce will to power. Protesters seek to exercise the power to define what counts as legitimate or authentic Christianity, Hinduism, or yoga and therefore relegate perceived others to outside the relevant tradition. The Christian yogaphobic position and the Hindu origins position both assume essentialist definitions of yoga in protest against its popularization in a struggle for the power to define what yoga really *is*. They denounce postural yogis for either compromising Christianity (the Christian yogaphobic position) or corrupting Hinduism (the Hindu origins position).

These protests are cases of a larger phenomenon: defining yoga with the aim of inciting fear of perceived others. Today, the dominant fear is that the popularization of yoga results in its infringement upon the boundaries of static religions. The politics of yoga is intimately tied to its religious associations, and it is necessary to critically examine attempts at defining yoga in terms of those associations for real-life consequences. Such an examination reveals that they support rifts in scholarship and in popular culture by reifying notions of the alien other.

In this chapter, I have called into question the definitions of yoga offered by the Christian yogaphobic position and the Hindu origins position. Their simplistic analyses, which are complicit with certain political and social agendas, function to perpetuate revisionist historical representations that do not accurately account for the dynamic history of yoga nor the experiences of many living, practicing yogis.

In their protests against the popularization of yoga, both positions betray truths about their subjectivity as participants in consumer culture, namely that individuals self-consciously exercise choice when it comes to worldviews and practices and the dominant cultural assumption that individuals should choose physical fitness products as parts of their regimens of self-development. Although opponents betray these truths, they do so unintentionally.

The history of yoga demonstrates that yoga functions as a source of a wide range of meanings and functions. Yoga has a long history whereby adherents of numerous religions, including Hindu, Jain, Buddhist, Christian, and New Age traditions, have constructed, deconstructed, and reconstructed it anew. Symbols, practices, and ideas vary across yoga studios and ashrams within South Asia alone, thus illustrating that the quest for the essence of yoga is an impossible task.

In the history of religions, there are no original ideas or practices, and there are no unchanging essences. Religious phenomena arise from continuous processes of syncretism, appropriation, and hybridization. Yoga is no exception. In short, the problem with any essentialist definition of yoga remains: Who's to say which, if any, yogis have it all wrong?

Conclusion

Its detractors say that classes are too big, that there isn't a lot of advanced alignment breakdowns, that the exclamation HAA-sss isn't the way you are supposed to breathe. He mimics a naysayer, sniffing: "Oh, that's not yoga!" He laughs and shrugs, a wordless: Who's to say what is yoga?

—MARY BILLARD on an interview with postural yoga
entrepreneur Greg Gumucio (2010a)

THE PREVALENT CONTEMPORARY vision of yoga derives from two recent historical forces: the rise to dominance of global market capitalism and the widespread diffusion of consumer culture. In the popular imagination, yoga connotes spandex-clad, perspiring, toned bodies brought together in rooms filled with yoga mats and engaged in a fitness regimen. And this despite the historical reality that, far from representing a static and homogenous essence, yoga is a symbol that has dramatically shifted in meaning across social contexts, including contemporary ones.

Despite its heterogeneity, the debate over what yoga *is* has persisted and has had scholarly and cultural consequences as well as political and economic ones. In my attempt to account for postural yoga's global diffusion and popularization by locating its intersections with consumer culture, I continuously came across attempts on the part of both postural yoga proponents and opponents to define what yoga *is* by locating some monolithic "center" or essence, even though contemporary popularized varieties of postural yoga are no less specific to their contexts within consumer culture than preceding varieties of modern and premodern yoga systems were specific to their relevant social contexts. Given the vast history of yoga and the degree to which it has been morphed (or mangled, as some critics of certain yoga systems would suggest) into various things over time, I suggest its context sensitivity serves as an important model of how cultural products adapt to shifting contexts. In my view, the most important lesson from the history of yoga and the divergent meanings attached to it is yoga's malleability (literally, the capacity to be bent into new shapes without breaking) in the hands of human beings.

Recent scholarship on premodern yoga tends to emphasize the significant role of social contexts in shaping premodern yoga systems and points to its heterogeneity based on empirical data rather than construct visions of yoga as homogenous and static. Scholars have spent much effort understanding the contextualized nature of premodern yoga by attending to the particularities of different systems and asking how they vary based on social context (I cited numerous such studies in Chapter One; see, e.g., Davidson 2002; Chapple 2003; White 2006; Bronkhorst 2007; Samuel 2008; White 2009; Chapple 2011; Wallace 2011; Larson 2012; White 2012). By the end of the first millennium c.e., yoga proponents in different Hindu, Buddhist, and Jain traditions systematized yoga in definitive terms. Following the twelfth-century Muslim incursions into South Asia and the establishment of Islam as a South Asian religion, even Sufis appropriated elements of yoga. Although there were countless attempts to define yoga leading up to the modern period, there was no homogenous center around which all yoga proponents and practitioners oriented themselves. Therefore, it was more accurate to identify it as heterogeneous in practice and characteristic of the doctrinally diverse premodern culture of South Asia than with any particular religio-philosophical tradition, Hindu or otherwise. Images of yoga from the premodern world included but were not limited to philosopher-ascetics turning inward in pursuit of salvation through realization of the true self, ecstatic *bhaktas* or devotees turning outward in pursuit of divine union with Krishna, and sinister villains channeling bodily energy in pursuit of sexual pleasure or political power. In short, premodern yoga was culturally South Asian, but its content and aims could not be reified.

Social contexts were key to shaping premodern yoga systems; hence, Vesna Wallace suggests that "the socio-political environments of the Yogic and Tantric practices at some point became replicated in the structures of these practices and determined their social values," and "certain social principles that guide religious practices can become transformed and in some cases even nullified in response to historical and sociopolitical contexts" (Wallace 2011: 336).

Recent scholarship on modern yoga also emphasizes the significant role of social contexts in shaping modern yoga systems and points to its heterogeneity rather than envisions it as homogenous and static. Modern yoga systems, including postural yoga ones, bear little resemblance to the yoga systems that preceded them, since modern yoga acclimated to shifting contexts. Yet, as yoga became a transnational product, nineteenth- and twentieth-century thinkers persistently attempted to define yoga by locating its center or essence, a constant that could be found in modern yoga systems but could also be traced back to yoga's so-called origins.

In my discussion of the early history of modern yoga in Chapter Two, I suggested that perhaps the most important lesson from the early history of modern yoga is the tradition's malleability, although, with all of the divergences that made up that history, the data reinforced a social pattern: Proponents of modern yoga, until the second half of the twentieth century, were countercultural, elite, or scandalous. Nevertheless, proponents varied from Indian ascetic renouncers, to turn-of-the-century American appropriators of tantra, to Transcendentalists and proponents of a variety of forms of metaphysical religion, to Hindu reformers and Indian nationalists, and to physical culture advocates. All of these groups defined yoga differently, although those who insisted on the bifurcation between what they perceived as true yoga or raja yoga and corrupt yoga or hatha yoga, such as Swami Vivekananda and Helena Blavatsky, made the most notable attempts to dogmatically assert its essence.

Scholars have offered valuable studies that further our understanding of the contextualized nature of modern yoga and, more specifically, postural yoga (I cited numerous such studies in preceding chapters; see, e.g., Sjoman 1996; Alter 2004; de Michelis 2004; Strauss 2005; Singleton 2010). In the current study, I have sought to expand the contextualist history of yoga to include a new chapter in that narrative, a chapter that seriously considers popularized varieties of postural yoga as what can serve as bodies of religious practice. I suggested that such yoga systems are products specific to the context of consumer culture, and I brought critical scrutiny to bear on the religious expressions peculiar to those systems. Rather than write off popularized varieties of postural yoga as mere "commodities" or "borrowings," I suggested that they share with other yoga systems the quality of being specific to a certain social context, and just because that social context is consumer culture does not mean that they do not have idiosyncratic meanings and functions beyond utilitarian or hedonistic ones.

In the late 1960s, yoga underwent popularization in many urban areas across the world, and attempts to define it according to a center or essence went hand in hand with that process. But proponents defined yoga in ways no longer opposed to the prevailing cultural norms of the masses. In fact, the second half of the twentieth century marked a new phase of development in the history of modern yoga. In consumer culture, modern yoga was no longer a countercultural, scandalous, or elite movement but was a part of transnational popular culture. Popularization did not happen equally everywhere. For example, in more conservative sectors of American and European cultures, residual cultural norms that opposed experimentation with anything deemed to have non-Christian origins prevented the popularization of yoga. But in many urban areas across the globe, postural yoga became increasingly accessible and commonly consumed among the general populace as its proponents established continuity with consumer culture.

New ways of defining yoga, primarily through the construction and marketing of sundry yoga brands, made possible continuity with consumer culture and therefore popularization. Yoga became subject to branding processes as economies in urban areas increasingly shifted toward the production and consumption of customized products based on individual consumers' desires and needs. Popular yoga brands varied in many ways—consider the more gentle approach of Anusara Yoga compared to the more onerous approach of Bikram Yoga—but they all signified the dominant physical and psychological self-developmental desires and needs of consumer society.

Yoga brands also reflected a response to transnational developments, not a transplantation of a bounded system from one static culture to another. In other words, yoga brands represented a response to transnational popular consumer desires and needs, not reified Indian or American cultural tendencies, hence the popularization of yoga in urban areas in India, Japan, Western Europe, Iran, North America, and other regions.

Two first-generation yoga entrepreneurs, B. K. S. Iyengar and Swami Muktananda, served as exempla in Chapter Four of first-generation yoga brands. Iyengar and Muktananda constructed Iyengar Yoga and Siddha Yoga respectively. Iyengar selected from the unbranded yoga system of Tirumalai Krishnamacharya and mass-marketed a postural yoga brand that defined yoga in terms of modern conceptions of physical fitness, biomechanics, and well-being, all of which dominated the self-developmental discourse of consumer culture. Muktananda selected from the unbranded yoga systems as prescribed by his guru, Nityananda, and as found in Vedanta and Kashmir Shaivism. He then mass-marketed a soteriological yoga brand that established some but less continuity with consumer culture, defining yoga in terms of modern democratic values, self-realization, transcendent states, and devotion.

John Friend served as an example of a second-generation yoga entrepreneur. He selected from Iyengar Yoga and Siddha Yoga and subsequently introduced, elaborated, and fortified the Anusara Yoga brand. By successfully constructing a brand that defined yoga in terms of a modern conception of health, the affirmation of life, lightheartedness, and community, he succeeded in the competitive global yoga market. He also served as an example of how gaffes in brand image management—Friend was perceived as transgressing Anusara Yoga ethical guidelines—can damage a yoga brand image and how the success of a yoga brand has as much to do with defining yoga in terms of its associations with particular persons as with particular values, methods, or discourses.

The cases of Iyengar Yoga, Siddha Yoga, and Anusara Yoga illustrated how, in different ways, yoga brands are saturated with meaning insofar as how they define yoga signifies what different segments of consumer society deem valuable. They also illustrated that contemporary consumers self-consciously choose products and services based on what they consider the most effective and accessible path—or brand—to get there.

Although many modern yoga brands were diffused throughout the world in the late twentieth century, including Hindu, Buddhist, and even Jain varieties, the most successful attempts at diffusion occurred when proponents consistently established continuity with consumer cultural trends. These were the postural yoga proponents. Their successful popularization of readily consumable postural yoga products and services reflected a phenomenon in the history of religions as a whole in which religious individuals and institutions continuously define their wares anew in response to particular social contexts. Despite the fact that it reflected that general phenomenon, there were a number of unique qualities of postural yoga that reflected its continuity with consumer culture. Examples of where continuity between the most popularized varieties and consumer culture occurred included the following: a nondualist metaphysics concerned with the union of mind–body–spirit, a concern with enhancing the body as a part of self-development, an approach to healing and resolving suffering that privileges modern biomedical discourse, and the disciplining of desire for the sake of health and beauty, again defined according to modern conceptions.

Although there was no doubt that many of the ways in which yoga proponents marketed postural yoga reflected continuity with consumer culture, yoga marketers and consumers also reflected the fact that, even in the socioeconomic context of market capitalism, not all consumption is the consumption of material goods for hedonistic or utilitarian aims. To demonstrate the nonhedonistic or utilitarian dimensions of postural yoga, I uncovered evidence of it being defined in religious ways everywhere, from popular magazines and websites to strip-mall yoga studios. Examples included opponents of regulatory attempts in Texas defining yoga as "spiritual"; postural yogis refusing to use what were perceived as overly commodified yoga mats, since "the ecstasy of yoga can't be contained in a mat"; and Christians establishing yoga systems through which one could become "closer to Christ." In fact, branding yoga products and making them sacred were not incompatible but rather were analogous processes. In the same way that religious individuals and institutions demarcate the sacred, yoga entrepreneurs demarcate a brand by making it special, by setting it apart, which often involves some attempt at locating a center or essence to yoga.

Yoga proponents were not the only ones providing essentialist definitions of yoga. Those privileging an outsider perspective at the exclusion of insider perspectives often defined postural yoga in ways that limited what type of yoga counted as legitimate, religious, ethical, or compatible with what were deemed authentic Christianity, authentic Hinduism, or even authentic yoga itself.

Carrette and King suggested that postural yoga is nothing more than a capitalist enterprise, in contrast to premodern yoga, which they defined as that which "involves a reorientation *away* from the concerns of the individual and towards an appreciation of the wider social and cosmic dimensions of our existence" (2005: 121). Advocates of the Christian yogaphobic position and the Hindu origins position both made the greatest efforts toward imposing essentialist definitions upon yoga in protest against its popularization. They denounced postural yogis for either compromising what was perceived as authentic Christianity (the Christian yogaphobic position) or corrupting what was perceived as authentic Hinduism (the Hindu origins position).

One of the most controversial American cases involving definitions of yoga as essentially religious and, more specifically, Hindu involved the debate over yoga in Encinitas, California, public schools as some parents, working in conjunction with the National Center for Law & Policy (NCLP), campaigned to remove recently introduced postural yoga classes from public schools, arguing that yoga promotes Hinduism.[1] Similar debates have occurred in India, where some members of the Indian Parliament have regularly and frequently attempted to make postural yoga compulsory in schools as a part of physical, not religious, education. Such attempts have infuriated some Indian Muslims, however, who suggest that teaching yoga in schools is a part of a Hindu nationalist agenda and tantamount to religious—specifically, Hindu—indoctrination. In October 2013, the Supreme Court heard arguments in favor of making yoga a compulsory part of physical education in Indian public schools. The Court hesitated to agree with arguments in favor of compulsory yoga in schools and asked, "Can we be asking all the schools to have one period for yoga classes every day when certain minority institutions may have reservations against it?" (Anand 2013). The Court concluded it should hear from minority groups arguing against making yoga compulsory before making a decision.

There were also regulatory attempts based on the assumption that yoga is not by definition essentially religious in several American states, including Texas, Connecticut, Washington, and Missouri. Threats of regulation included imposing sales taxes on yoga classes and regulating yoga teacher training programs. Protesters against regulation suggested that yoga is by definition "spiritual"; some of them even cited their First Amendment rights to free exercise of religion.

I could go on and on providing examples of attempts to define yoga in ways that limit it to certain bounded categories of belief or behavior, such as "exercise," "spirituality," "religion," or "Hinduism," and accordingly outside of others, but I will add only one more to the list. In 2002, there was a transnational public outcry in response to Bikram Choudhury and the school for which he is Founder, Chairman, and CEO, Bikram's Yoga College of India (BYCI). He and his school had attempted to enforce copyrights over Bikram Yoga's sequence of twenty-six postures on yoga studios claiming to teach Bikram Yoga but not conforming to the BYCI's standards (Figs. 7.1–7.4). Allison Fish suggests this case serves as an example of how the global market for yoga, given the difficulty in locating and defining it, has consequences for how open source and Intellectual Property Rights (IPRs) are defined and how information management strategies emerge (2006). The case, indeed, called for different participants to take a stand

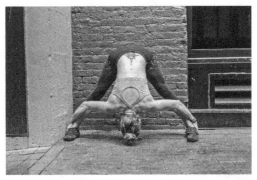

FIGURE 7.1 Bikram Yoga teacher Kirsten Greene in the *dandayamana-bibhaktapada paschimotthana asana* (standing separate leg stretching posture).

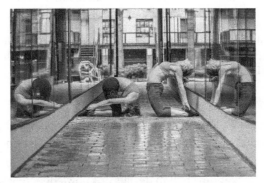

FIGURE 7.2 Kirsten Greene (left) in the deepest forward bend of the Bikram Yoga postural sequence, *sasanga asana* (rabbit posture), and Bikram Yoga teacher Sabine Hagen (right) in the deepest backward bend of the Bikram Yoga postural sequence, *ustra asana* (camel posture).

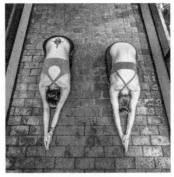

FIGURE 7.3 Kirsten Greene (left) and Sabine Hagen (right) in the *ardha-kurma asana* (half tortoise posture).

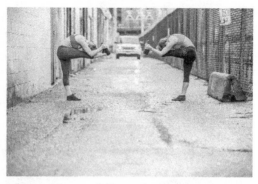

FIGURE 7.4   Sabine Hagen (left) and Kirsten Greene (right) in the *dandayamana-janushira asana* (standing head to knee posture).

[Figures 7.1–7.4] Kirsten Greene and Sabine Hagen are both certified teachers of Bikram Yoga. They trained with Bikram Choudhury, Rajashree Choudhury, and several senior teachers in the Bikram Yoga Teacher Training program in Los Angeles, California and currently serve as Bikram Yoga teachers in Squamish, British Columbia. Above, they are pictured in some of the onerous postures of the Bikram Yoga twenty-six postural sequence. Photographed by Michael Petrachenko. (Images courtesy of Kirsten Greene.)

with regard to how to define and categorize new conceptualizations or applications of what are popularly considered "preexisting materials" or "traditional knowledge." Contemporary entrepreneurs are perpetually branding and packaging such materials or knowledge in new ways for the sake of attracting consumers.

Choudhury and the BYCI were involved in two United States federal court lawsuits, which were settled out of court under nondisclosure agreements, and they threatened many more around the world (Fish 2006: 192).[2] In 2012, however, the United States Copyright Office concluded that the copyrights issued to Choudhury and the BYCI were issued in error (Federal Register 2012): Neither Choudhury and the BYCI nor any other individual or organization could copyright yoga postures or their sequences. In response to the question of whether "the selection and arrangement of preexisting exercises, such as yoga poses" are copyrightable, the Office answered with a definitive "no" (Office of the Federal Register 2012: 37607).[3] The refusal to grant copyrights to yoga posture "compilations" or sequences is based on the idea that "exercise is not a category of authorship" (Office of the Federal Register 2012: 37607); therefore, it is based on the assumption that postural yoga, by definition, is "exercise." The Copyright Office offered the following assessment of claims to copyrights of yoga sequences and, more specifically, the claims made by Choudhury:

> In the view of the Copyright Office, a selection, coordination, or arrangement of exercise movements, such as a compilation of yoga poses, may be precluded from registration as a functional system or process in cases where the particular movements and the order in which they are to be performed are said to result in improvements in one's health or physical or mental condition. *See, e.g, Open Source Yoga Unity v. Choudhury,* 2005 WL 756558, *4, 74 U.S.P.Q.2d 1434 (N.D. Cal. 2005) ("Here, Choudhury claims that he arranged the asanas in a manner that was both aesthetically pleasing and in a way that he believes is best designed to improve the practitioner's health."). While such a functional system or process may be aesthetically appealing, it is nevertheless uncopyrightable subject matter. (Office of the Federal Register 2012: 37607)

In this case, the Copyright Office determined whether sequences of yoga postures were copyrightable based on a definition of postural yoga as "exercise," since its aims included "health."

The Government of the United States was not the only one to respond to Choudhury and the BYCI's efforts to establish and enforce copyrights. In part as an act of resistance to Choudhury and the BYCI's attempts to claim ownership of certain postural yoga sequences, the Indian government-run Traditional Knowledge Digital Library (TKDL) created a database of thirteen hundred yoga postures believed to be documented in ancient Indian texts (Sinha 2011). The Indian government's agenda is akin to that of proponents of the Hindu origins position. Whereas proponents of the Hindu origins position seek to prevent what they perceive as the inequitable profiteering off knowledge they perceive as belonging to Hinduism, the Indian government seeks to prevent the profiteering off that which it perceives as belonging to India. And, like the United States Copyright Office, the Government of India resisted corporate claims of ownership by offering up a legal definition of yoga as a "physical discipline" aimed at improving "health." However, in a dramatically different move from that of the United States, the Government of India also offered a legal definition of yoga that located its origins in the ancient text, Patanjali's *Yoga Sutras*:

Yoga is one of the six systems of Vedic philosophy. Maharishi Patanjali, rightly called 'The Father of Yoga,' compiled and refined various aspects of Yoga systematically in his 'Yoga Sutras' (aphorisms). He advocated the eight folds path of Yoga, popularly known as 'Ashtanga Yoga,' for all-round development of human beings. They are: Yama, Niyama, Asana, Pranayama, Pratyahara, Dharana, Dhyana and Samadhi. These components advocate certain restraints and observances, physical discipline, breath regulations, restraining the sense organs, contemplation, meditation and samadhi. These steps are believed to have a potential for improvement of physical health by enhancing circulation of oxygenated blood in the body, retraining the sense organs thereby inducing tranquility and serenity of mind. The practice of Yoga prevents psychosomatic disorders and improves an individual's resistance and ability to endure stressful situations. (Department of AYUSH 2010)

The continuous attempts to define yoga in ways that limit its meanings and functions are reminiscent of contemporary attempts to define other cultural formations, such as Christianity or Islam. Consider the recent effort to and success in trademarking Islam in Pakistan.[4] In 1993, there was a judicial decision that, for the first time in history, provided a detailed government definition of Islam. The presiding judge declared that the symbols and rites of Islam, such as the profession of faith and mosques, were intellectual property that were subject to copyrighting, although he failed to articulate how to establish claims of ownership. Consequently, any individual or institution that "improperly" recited the profession of faith or named a building a mosque was using copyrighted material without permission and was liable to legal penalties. Carl Ernst suggests:

The implications of this decision are breathtaking. Not only is a religion being defined as a commodity or piece of property, which the judge actually compared to Coca-Cola, but also the courts— not religious communities—are entitled to decide what is essential to any religion. Moreover, in this decision the limits of Islam are being defined in relation to a modern sectarian group. Current Pakistani passports now require professed Muslim citizens to sign a declaration that they adhere to the finality of the prophethood of Muhammad—that is, that they are not Ahmadis. Such an outcome (reminiscent of oaths of orthodox interpretation of Holy Communion during the Protestant Reformation) can only be imagined as a result of very recent local history. (Ernst 2003: 205)

The debate amounts to the question of whether the meaning of *Islam* should be restricted to the level of "minimum conformity with the expectations of a particular Muslim community" (Ernst 2003: 206). Ernst retorts:

> But the problem with any authoritative definition of religion remains the same: Who is entitled to define Islam? In any society in the world today, religious pluralism is a sociological fact. If one group claims authority over all the rest, demanding their allegiance and submission, this will be experienced as the imposition of power through religious rhetoric. (Ernst 2003: 206)

Likewise, the problem with any authoritative definition of yoga is that there are no responsible ways to determine who holds the exclusive authority to define it, and any attempt to claim that authority amounts to a fierce imposition of power. All participants in the ongoing debate over defining yoga, determining who should "do" yoga, and deciding whether or not to exercise state control over its distribution, find themselves forced to address the question, "What is yoga?" Regulation of something, whether by a religious or state institution, requires a definition of the thing targeted.

Despite the historical reality that yoga has always been a vexed and contested concept and has always been contextual, there are continuous attempts to define yoga. Many of the attempts to define postural yoga as essentially religious—most often, as Hindu—or as essentially nonreligious (or nonspiritual)—most often, as mere exercise or commodification— betray a tendency to ignore the more complex perspectives of many insiders to postural yoga. In any serious analysis of postural yoga, privileging outsider perspectives results in an account that does not take seriously contemporary practitioners' experiences of or desires for yoga. How then could it claim to adequately define, explain, or even describe postural yoga? For many contemporary postural yogis, yoga is like religious institutions and organizations insofar as it is assumed to be beyond the reach of a legal definition or one that ignores its meanings and functions, which are believed to transcend hedonistic fulfillments or utilitarian gains. At the same time, many of them think of postural yoga as the best form of exercise and love yoga pants because they think they make their butts look good. The debate over regulation, therefore, brings questions to light about how one would formulate a definition of postural yoga and if that would even be possible if one intends to account for *all* postural yogis. Such an attempt to define postural yoga would amount to identifying a bounded tradition of symbols, practices, values, and ideas, which in reality vary across postural yoga studios and the individuals inside of them.

The tendency to search for the center or essence of a complex human phenomenon, such as a body of religious practice, in order to locate it within or outside of bounded categories has a long history in the study of religions. Friedrich Schleiermacher's effort to locate an essence in Christianity serves as a paragon of that tendency. In 1830, Schleiermacher suggested:

> The only pertinent way of discovering the peculiar essence of any particular faith and reducing it as far as possible to a formula is by showing the element which remains constant throughout the most diverse religious affections within this same communion, while it is absent from analogous affections within other communions. (Schleiermacher 1999 [1830]: 52)

In short, Schleiermacher suggests that the scholar should locate the unchanging center of a religious complex around which all alternating qualities revolve.[5]

Reacting against such tendencies in the history of the study of religion, Jonathan Z. Smith (1993 [1978]) suggests that scholars avoid the tendency to "lay prime emphasis upon congruency and conformity" (293). He suggests that scholars instead direct inquiry toward exploring "the dimensions of incongruity that exist in religious materials" (293). On defining *Hinduism*, some scholars have pointed out that Hinduism is still understood through fiercely Orientalist lenses that are often combined with a revisionist history that does not take account of the history of colonial India and Orientalism. Richard King, for example, criticizes essentialist accounts, suggesting that "the postulation of a single, underlying *religious* unity called 'Hinduism' requires a highly imaginative act of historical reconstruction" (King 1999: 110). More specifically, he targets two forms of Orientalist discourse that result in authoritative and essentializing approaches to what are in fact complex and incongruous phenomena:

Simplistically speaking, we can speak of two forms of Orientalist discourse, the first, generally antagonistic and confident in European superiority, the second, generally affirmative, enthusiastic and suggestive of Indian superiority in certain key areas. Both forms of Orientalism, however, make essentialist judgments that foster an overly simplistic and homogenous conception of Indian culture. (King 1999: 116)

In place of Orientalist discourses, King suggests scholars take "a non-essentialist approach that draws particular attention to the ruptures and discontinuities, the criss-crossing patterns and 'family resemblances' that are usually subsumed by unreflective and essentialist usage" (King 110).[6] King points to anthropologist Gabriella Eichinger Ferro-Luzzi's (1991) work, which applies a family resemblance approach to Hinduism, suggesting that scholars should retain the term *Hinduism* but understand it as a "polythetic-prototypical" concept. It is *polythetic* because it is radically heterogeneous, and it is *prototypical* because people use it to refer to a particular idealized construct. The prototypical qualities include both what are common among Hindus (e.g., temple worship or the worship of deities such as Shiva and Krishna) and what have prestige among Hindus, especially elite Hindus (e.g., brahmanical concepts of *dharma* or *advaita*) (Ferro-Luzzi 1991: 192).

More recently, Wendy Doniger critiques the many attempts to limit what counts as Hindu by defining Hinduism in terms of an essence or center. Doniger suggests there is "no central something" to what is commonly referred to by the essentializing term *Hinduism*. She and other scholars have suggested ways to move forward in the study of Hindu traditions without limiting what counts as legitimate or authentic by offering *polythetic approaches* to defining Hinduism, approaches that "[identify] a cluster of qualities each of which is important but not essential to Hinduism" (Doniger 2009: 28).[7] So every quality is not present in every case of what one might categorize as *Hinduism*, and, additionally, whatever cluster of qualities one identifies at any given time and place is in fact "constantly changing" (Doniger 2009: 29). The person who adopts the polythetic approach therefore must be prepared for changes with shifting contexts.

Although today the popular imagination relies on such distinguishing and reified categories as *Hindu* and *yoga* to think about what are perceived as identifiable, bounded traditions, those terms have been far more fluid,

contested, and unstable in their applications throughout history. And anyone interested in approaching postural yoga in a way that accounts for
its rich variation and context sensitivity as well as insider and outsider
perspectives and that avoids revisionist histories must resist the tendency
to locate a claimed center or essence around which all postural yoga practice revolves. The evidence discussed in the current study suggests that
attempts to locate the "peculiar essence" of yoga and, more specifically,
of postural yoga consistently fail to do so in a way that is consistent with
both the historical record and with all or even most insiders' experiences.

This study has identified a number of qualities that at different times
and places have functioned as the "center" of yoga, although that center
has been at the "periphery" for yogis at other times and places. The history of postural yoga demonstrates that yoga functions as a source of a
wide range of meanings and functions; therefore, I suggest that a polythetic approach is the most effective for understanding it.

The person who adopts a polythetic approach to understanding the
history of yoga understands that to apply such conceptual constructs as
yoga, modern yoga, or *postural yoga* to data accumulating around the term
yoga is not to imply that each is monolithic or static. Rather, they are living, dynamic traditions; hence the divergences between figures like the
sexologist Ida C. Craddock and the tycoon Pierre Bernard, the physical
fitness giants Iyengar and Choudhury, or the tantric entrepreneur John
Friend and the evangelical Christian Brooke Boon.

At best, one might suggest that *postural yoga* refers to a collection of
complex data made up of a congeries of figures, institutions, ideas, and
practical paths involving mental or physical techniques—most commonly
meditative, breathing, or postural exercises. It is believed to resolve the
problem of suffering and to improve health, both defined in modern
terms. Postural yoga often betrays a desire to repair what is perceived as
an imbalance of "body–mind–soul." Finally, it is tied to mythologies about
the historical transmission of yogic knowledge, accumulating around a
transnational community that has engaged in and transmitted what participants call *yoga*—and sometimes refuse to call *yoga*—since the twentieth century.

Much of what makes up the contemporary postural yoga world is
specific to its social context: consumer culture. Therefore, much of what
we say about it betrays more about that cultural context than about any
monolithic conception of yoga. As discussed in preceding chapters, many
contemporary postural yogis maintain an ontological position that sees

the body's enhancement as key to self-development and are primarily concerned with practical muscle-building and stretching postures deemed paths to health. They often aim primarily at a modern notion of physical health, although many postural yogis also see *health* as encapsulating psychological or even spiritual well-being.

Furthermore, the historical deposit demonstrates that postural yoga systems, in all of their various manifestations, cannot be judged as authentic or inauthentic relative to one another or to ancient or so-called classical yoga traditions. They must be understood instead in terms of the collective and divergent meanings and functions their practitioners attribute to them. According to the history of postural yoga, those include the sacralization of the body, the mystico-erotic union with divinity, pleasure, the path to self-actualization or self-realization, as well as modern notions of health, beauty, sex appeal, and fitness. In the postural yoga world, *yoga* can signify all of these meanings and functions.

One postural yogi's center is another's periphery. If one person's center is another's periphery in the world of yoga, then how should one define it—and should one attempt to do so at all? The only responsible way to define yoga is to do so in pluralist terms through a polythetic approach. Any attempt to locate a center or essence of yoga would fail to include at least some of the wide variety of the postural yoga insiders discussed in this study, and, as implied by one postural yogi's shrug at naysayers to *his* rendition of yoga, "Who's to say what is yoga?"

Notes

1. The Jain tradition is a predominantly South Asian religion grounded in the dualist belief that the natural world is distinct from the spiritual one and ritual discipline aimed at an ascetic ideal whereby one conquers the natural world by shutting down all physical and psychological needs and desires. In fact, the term *Jain* is derived from the Sanskrit term *jina* or "conqueror." *Jina* is a title ascribed to twenty-four great ascetic teachers who are featured in a number of myths in which they "conquer" their own needs and desires through withdrawal from bodily action and social engagement and through the cultivation of nonviolence (*ahimsa*) toward all living beings. There are two major Jain sects: Digambara or "sky-clad" and Shvetambara or "white-clad." Their names refer to whether or not their fully initiated monastics remain nude or wear white robes. Within each, there are several subsects, including a Digambara Terapanth and a Shvetambara Terapanth. In this study, *Terapanth* refers to the Shvetambara Terapanth exclusively. The Terapanth emerged in eighteenth-century Rajasthan as a Shvetambara reform movement aimed toward the return of the Jain tradition to what were perceived as its founder's, Mahavira's, original teachings. Although still organizationally headquartered in Rajasthan, in the late twentieth century the Terapanth developed into a global movement aimed toward the dissemination of Jain thought and practice. For a more detailed discussion of Mahaprajna and the Terapanth, see Chapter Three.

2. On the term *postural yoga*, see de Michelis 2004 and Singleton 2010. See also my discussion below on yoga categorization. As I will suggest throughout this study, postural yoga systems, although they share a concern with posture and breathing, make up a complex and highly contested phenomenon that can take many forms and have various meanings and functions for its practitioners.

3. *Muni* or "silent one," a title that alludes to the monastic withdrawal from society, is the most common title ascribed to Terapanth male monastics and is commonly used in other South Asian monastic traditions.

4. As a practical application of the Jain vow of *ahimsa* or "nonviolence" to all living beings, Terapanth monastics wear the mouth-shield to prevent the undesired inhalation and consequent destruction of organisms in the air.

5. *Samana* is derived from the Sanskrit word *shramana*, which means "striver" and is used as an epithet for world-renouncers in South Asia. It is used in the sense of one who "strives" for release from the cycle of rebirth.

6. The respect I have for my parents, Linda and Vikash Jain, for traversing the socio- and ethno-cultural spaces rarely traversed before by marrying one another in 1974 is immeasurable.

7. For examples, see Qvarnström 1998: 47 and Olivelle 1993: 244–246. Qvarnström discusses this process with regard to the Jain literary tradition in the medieval period of South Asian history. Olivelle discusses this topic as it applies to Brahmanical religious systems or what we have come to call *Hinduism* in South Asia.

8. I capitalize yoga only when following the custom of a specific institutionalized yoga movement under consideration (for example, Siddha Yoga).

CHAPTER 1

1. Citing Arnold van Gennep on rites of passage, Elizabeth de Michelis argues that a class in Modern Postural Yoga (throughout this book, I use the less reificatory term, *postural yoga*) functions as a "healing ritual of secular religion" (de Michelis 2004: 252; on rites of passage, see van Gennep 1965 [1908]). Also citing Victor Turner, de Michelis argues that the postural yoga class functions as a "liminal space" (de Michelis 2004: 252; on ritual liminality, see Turner, Victor 2008 [1969]). The practitioner undergoes both physical and psychological transformations and healing before being reintroduced to "everyday life" (de Michelis 2004: 252–257). For more on the ritual dimensions of postural yoga, see Chapter Five.

2. I use *sacred* here in the broad Durkheimian sense of that which is set apart from the ordinary or mundane. Émile Durkheim suggests the sacred is antagonistic to the profane (Durkheim 2001 [1912]). The distinction between what is sacred and what is profane can only be defined by their heterogeneity (Durkheim 2001 [1912]: 38). On the sacred dimension of postural yoga, see Chapter Five.

3. For sources on the invention of modern yoga, see Chapters Two and Three. On the invention of modern yoga postures in particular, I discuss Mark Singleton's *Yoga Body* (2010) in Chapter Three.

4. The English translation of the invocation provided by the official B. K. S. Iyengar website is as follows: "Let us bow before the noblest of sages Patanjali, who gave yoga for serenity and sanctity of mind, grammar for clarity and purity of

speech and medicine for perfection of health. Let us prostrate before Patanjali, an incarnation of Adisesa, whose upper body has a human form, whose arms hold a conch and a disc, and who is crowned by a thousand-headed cobra" (Ramamani Iyengar Memorial Yoga Institute 2009b).

5. Singleton, however, points out that there is nothing in the verses that Jois cites that pertains in any way to either the sequences or their individual postures (Singleton 2010: 221–222, n. 4).

6. The argument for yoga's origins in the Indus Valley Civilization assumes that the Civilization has direct ties to later South Asian religious complexes, an issue that is hotly debated. Positions take four forms based on the perceived cultural interaction between the Indus Valley Civilization and Indo-Europeans. First, scholars argue that Indo-Europeans invaded India and conquered the Indus Valley Civilization. Second, scholars argue that the Indo-Europeans gradually migrated into India and settled among those who lived there. Third, scholars argue that the Vedic people were indigenous to India. Finally, scholars argue that the Vedic people were indigenous to India and were a part of the Indus Valley Civilization (for a summary of these four theories, see Doniger 2009: 85–102; for a discussion of these theories' historical plausibility and political dimensions, see Samuel 2008: 2–8, 19; Doniger 2009: 85–102).

7. See Chapter Two.

8. See Chapters Three, Four, Five, and Six.

9. The author of the *Bhagavad Gita* states that those "who have stopped the movements of breathing in (*prāṇa*) and breathing out (*apāna*) are devoted to *prāṇāyāma*)" (*Bhagavad Gita* 4:29, quoted in Bronkhorst 2007: 26). Likewise, the author of the *Yoga Sutras* states that pranayama entails "cutting off the movement of breathing out and breathing in" (*Yoga Sutras* 2:49, quoted in Bronkhorst 2007: 26–27).

10. On the Pashupati Seal and other seals from Indus Valley Civilization sites, see Fairservis 1975: 274–77; Hiltebeitel 1978: 767–779; McEvilley 1981; and Srinivasan 1984.

11. The most widely cited characteristics are the headdress, the posture, the multiple faces, and the presence of animals (Srinivasan 1984: 78–83).

12. On the absence of *yoga* in ancient Brahmanical contexts, Bronkhorst cites Monika Shee (1986: 204). Shee, in turn, cites Klaus Ruping (1977: 88) and Joachim Friedrich Sprockhoff (1976: 1–2).

13. Johannes Bronkhorst cites Jonathan Silk (1997; 2000), who suggests that the term *yoga* makes a late appearance in the "postcanonical" Buddhist literature, and Robert Williams (1963), who suggests that the early Jain sources use the term *yoga* but in an entirely idiosyncratic sense.

14. The ideals of modern postural yoga include contemporary female ideals, and, in fact, women are often disproportionately represented in modern

postural yoga milieus. However, Samuel argues that the idealization of male celibacy in both Brahmanical and Buddhist traditions has "destructive consequences for women," since "women have an ambivalent and difficult relationship to a social and ideological order constructed around the supremacy of certain kinds of men" (Samuel 2008: 188–189). Laurie L. Patton suggests that the mention of female ascetics in some Brahmanical texts might change the male "warrior-ascetic prototype" (2011: 316–317). She cites a number of studies that evaluate the possibility that there might have been ways of thinking about yoga outside of the "model of male celibacy" (Patton cites Vanita 2003; Black 2007; Dhand 2007). Samuel cites additional scholarship on women in the yoga tradition (Findly 1985; Lindquist 2008) but suggests that no clear conclusions can be drawn from narratives about "real-life women or about gender relations at the time of their composition" (2011: 339). As Steven E. Lindquist (2008) suggests, the inclusion of women "within a larger cast of anomalous characters" serves as an "internal critique and development of the Brahmin worldview and less of a reflection of historical reality" (417) and points to the ways in which ascetic women are constructed in the narrative as masculinized women (421–422).

15. *Samnyasin* is a Sanskrit term derived from *samnyasa*, which means "renunciation of the world." It is a term Brahmanic Hindus have used to refer to those who fully renounce previously held conventional social identities and material possessions in favor of a path exclusively aimed toward spiritual purification and advancement.

16. For more on the reification of a notion of classical yoga, see Chapters Two and Six.

17. Samuel suggests that these innovations might have been a result of influences from previously existing Chinese traditions, though this argument is speculative (2008: 278–282).

18. On Jain appropriations of tantra, see Cort 1987: 238; Chapple 1998: 15; Dundas 1998; Cort 2000: 417; and Dundas 2000: 232. Jain appropriations of tantra are discussed in more detail below.

19. Advaita Vedanta traditions assimilated many Nath yoga texts into their own canon in the early eighteenth century (Bouy 1994). Many of the compilers of that canon were biased toward orthodoxy and therefore omitted some key transgressive aspects of Nath yoga (Mallinson 2007:10). A similar form of censorship occurred again in the construction of modern yoga (see Chapter Two). Jains, discussed in more detail below, also adopted aspects of hatha yoga while omitting those aspects that would have threatened Jain orthodoxy (Qvarnström, 1998: 37).

20. Such antinomian practices on the part of the Kula tradition included ritual copulation and the ingestion of nonvegetarian foods.

CHAPTER 2

1. For details on Craddock's life and system of yoga, I primarily rely on Schmidt 2010. See also Chappell 2010.

2. The term *fundamentalism* dates to the early twentieth century, when the Bible Institute of Los Angeles published a series of booklets called *The Fundamentals* (1910–1915), which were the impetus for a movement that came to be known as fundamentalism. Early fundamentalists denounced modern ideas about the study of culture, history, and religion and called for Christianity to return to what they considered its "fundamentals," including belief in the inerrancy of the Bible. Fundamentalists were especially reacting to the advancement of research on religions that brought into question the Christian exceptionalism that had dominated Western European and American cultures in the previous century and thus cultivated more research on non-Christian and non-Western religions. The term *fundamentalist* was eventually more broadly applied to institutions or individuals from any religion who seek a return to what they perceive as the unchanging essence or "fundamentals" of their religions (on *fundamentalisms*, see Marty and Appleby 1993–2004).

3. As a way of demonstrating the extent to which mainstream Americans identified the country as Christian, consider an 1892 United States Supreme Court decision in which the court ruled that "we find everywhere a clear recognition of the same truth... that this is a Christian nation" (*Church of the Holy Trinity v. United States* 1892).

4. Comstock and other members of his organization also harassed and pursued legal cases against Pierre Bernard and members of the Theosophical Society (both discussed below).

5. On esoteric tantric traditions, see Chapter One.

6. Seminal retention occurs in sexual intercourse when the man withholds ejaculation for as long as possible. On the topic of ritual sexual intercourse, the *Tantras* sometimes prescribed seminal retention.

7. As noted below, the physical techniques of yoga were less subject to such criticism when they became associated with physical fitness in the twentieth century.

8. For details on Bernard's life and system of yoga, I primarily rely on Urban 2000, Urban 2003, and Love 2010.

9. One of those disciples, Blanche de Vries, taught many students in New York and California, including those who sponsored B. K. S. Iyengar's first trip to the United States in 1956 (Love 2010: 339). I will return to Iyengar and his role in the popularization of yoga in proceeding chapters.

10. For details on Woodroffe's esoteric engagement with tantric yoga, I primarily rely on Taylor 2001.

11. Transcendentalism was a nineteenth-century American literary and philosophical movement that opposed mainstream intellectual culture, including its doctrinaire rationalism and privileging of Protestant Christianity. Transcendentalists believed that, by means of intuition rather than doctrine, one could achieve an ideal transcendent spiritual state. Transcendentalists were not against rational thought as a means to attaining knowledge, but they argued for the value of intuition as well. Intuition, they suggested, underlies religion in its various forms.

12. This view of yoga's development as beginning as an intellectual movement and then degenerating into physical practice has no ground in historical evidence (see Chapter One).

13. Madame Helena Blavatsky and Colonel Henry Steel Olcott founded the Theosophical Society in 1875 in New York City. It was a spiritualist organization made up of individuals who sought religious reform by means of synthesizing Asian and Western metaphysical traditions in a variety of ways. By 1901, it had five hundred active chapters in forty-two countries where it offered a religious option that was counter to mainstream orthodoxies.

14. Shankara (circa eighth or ninth century C.E.), the most famous expounder of advaita vedanta, a nondualist version of South Asian philosophy, and the most famous of South Asian philosophers, suggested that ignorance is a result of projection. In order to attain *jnana* or "knowledge" and, most importantly, knowledge of the *atman* or true "self," one must learn to discriminate—and therefore put a stop to projection—between what is the self and what is not the self. Knowledge is attained when one realizes the ontological identity of the self with *brahman*, the cosmic essence. Modern advaita vedanta began with nineteenth-century figures and movements in India and North America (these included Transcendentalists, the Theosophical Society, New Thought, Vivekananda and his Ramakrishna Mission and Vedanta Society) and continued to flourish in the twentieth century (representatives included Paramahansa Yogananda (1893–1952) and his Self-Realization Fellowship, Maharishi Mahesh Yogi (1918–2008) and his Transcendental Meditation, and the Integral Yoga Institute). For a recent comprehensive study of these figures and movements, see Goldberg 2010.

15. The 1893 World's Parliament of Religions was held as part of the World's Columbian Exposition. The aim was for the Parliament to be the first formal gathering of global religious representatives, and for the result to be a dialogue between those representatives (although many representatives from religious traditions, such as Sikh and Native American, as well as other indigenous traditions, were left out of the dialogue).

16. *Raja yoga* has had various other meanings in many medieval and precolonial yoga texts, including, for example, the tantric Hamsavilasa, in which the term refers to "ecstatic sensual rapture" (Vasudeva 2012: 242).

17. For more on Vivekananda's censorship of the life of Ramakrishna, see Chapter Six.

18. For a history of metaphysical religion in the United States, see Albanese 2007.

19. See Chapter One. See also Singleton's discussion of the absence of any direct lineage between the South Asian yoga tradition and modern yoga as posture practice (Singleton 2010: 29–33).

20. Though hatha yoga is the traditional source of postural yoga, equating them does not account for postural yoga's historical sources. Such an equation would also fail to account for the variety of methods and aims that hatha yoga systems themselves have embraced since their emergence in the tenth to eleventh centuries that are not present in postural yoga, from identification with the divine while remaining in the body to supernatural powers and other mundane objectives discussed in Chapter One.

21. De Michelis places these centers in the Modern Yoga category *Modern Psychosomatic Yoga (MPsY)* (de Michelis 2004: 189).

22. Singleton adds that the Ashtanga Vinyasa system of Jois directly developed out of Krishnamacharya's system, and various other contemporary popular forms, such as "power yoga," "vinyasa flow," and "power vinyasa," that emerged primarily in the United States since the 1990s also developed out of that system. Furthermore, the postural yoga of B. K. S. Iyengar, which is less aerobic than those systems developed by Jois and his students, directly developed out of Krishnamacharya's system (2010: 176–177).

23. As Sarah Strauss suggests, Sivananda's reliance on printed materials for the dissemination of his teachings was a break from the traditional transmission of yoga in the one-on-one guru–disciple relationship, which does not reach large numbers easily (Strauss 2005: 45).

CHAPTER 3

1. Richard Hittleman was the first to bring yoga to American television in 1961 through his series, *Yoga for Health.*

2. Peter Brent was the first to use the term *godmen* in an academic text. It first appeared in his *Godmen of India* (1972).

3. "The term 'lifestyle,'" according to Mike Featherstone, "is currently in vogue ...within the contemporary consumer culture it connotes individuality, self-expression, and a stylistic self-consciousness. One's body, clothes, speech, leisure pastimes, eating and drinking preferences, home, car, choice of holidays, etc. are to be regarded as indicators of the individuality of taste and sense of style of the owner/consumer" (Featherstone 2007: 81).

4. Not all such pluralization, as Berger points out, means increased choice. As an example of increased pluralization without increased choice, Berger describes the contemporary citizen who has to pay five different sets of taxes as opposed

to the subject of a traditional ruler who only has to pay one (Berger 1979: 15–16). There is also the problem of increased class stratification, resulting in poverty-stricken populations who cannot afford to choose products based on individual preferences. Choice in the area of consumption is more so a part of the lives of the economically privileged; hence the popularization of yoga is largely a middle- to upper-class phenomenon.

5. It is not as if choice did not exist in premodern societies, and the extent to which contemporary social actors exercise choice certainly varies on a broad spectrum, based largely on socioeconomic class, but Berger maintains that the range of choices of many modern persons is beyond the scope of anything found in a premodern society in which certainty was "taken-for-granted" even though it was not "total" (Berger 1979: 3, 9). Scholars have problematized the tendency to speak of any universal developmental sequence, arguing that certain nation-states do not fit into the same Western-defined developmental sequence of tradition–modernity–postmodernity (see, e.g., Featherstone and Lash 1995). Despite the accuracy of that criticism, Berger's analysis remains useful because it addresses the fact that technological and economic shifts since the Enlightenment have in some way affected almost all human societies such that choice, to one degree or another, has become more heterogeneous and frequent relative to the premodern period, especially among upper classes and in urban areas.

6. Frederic Jameson famously identifies the "cultural logic of late capitalism"— what I call "consumer culture"—as "postmodernism," or the rejection of any single metanarrative and the concomitant fragmentation and pluralization of choice (Jameson 1991).

7. Modern thought here is concomitant with *modernism*, certain philosophical and sociocultural qualities founded in the Enlightenment, including the privileging of reason and rational order; the emergence of the cognitive subject; the rise of modern science and emphasis on material progress through scientific technologies; realism and representation as the dominant purpose of aesthetics; the emergence of industrial capitalism; and separation of production and consumption (Firat and Venkatesh 1995: 240).

8. Andreas Huyssen uses the categories *high culture* and *mass culture* in place of *elite culture* and *pop culture* respectively (Huyssen 1986: viii, 57).

9. Jameson uses the example of aesthetic production to demonstrate that cultural production is no longer distinct from consumption.

10. An *ashram* is a South Asian center of monastic retreat for religious study and training, usually under the guidance of a guru.

11. Consider, as a further example, the title of an edited volume on the Hare Krishna Movement: *The Hare Krishna Movement: The Postcharismatic Fate of a Religious Transplant* (Bryant and Ekstrand 2004).

12. As a contemporary example of visibility without popularization, consider Scientology in the first decades of twenty-first-century American culture.

Although Scientology is highly visible, especially as a consequence of its associations with a number of popular celebrities, it remains on the fringes of mainstream society.

13. Although Vivekananda and his disciples had established Vedanta Society centers in major cities throughout the United States, many soon struggled to survive while others had to shut down. The yoga movement that would emerge in the early twentieth century and would have the most direct long-term influence was that of Yogananda's Self-Realization Fellowship. In 1937, the *Self-Realization* magazine reported that over 150,000 individuals had been initiated. Yet with Yogananda's death in 1952, this movement underwent downsizing from its peak of about 150 Self-Realization centers in the United States (Tweed and Prothero 1999: 162).

14. The fact that body-centered systems of yoga were not popularized in the United States and Western Europe until the 1960s may have also been in part because there were strict immigration restrictions to the United States and Western Europe, thus limiting the extent to which Indian yoga gurus could disseminate postural yoga beyond India.

15. According to de Michelis's *Modern Yoga* typology, Modern Denominational Yoga includes certain systems that developed as far back as the 1960s. Such systems are concerned with religious and philosophical doctrine and are often characterized by the following qualities: allegiance to a guru figure; strict organizational structure; high demands on members; not primarily concerned with yoga; and exclusivist attitudes toward other religious systems (de Michelis 2004: 189). Relatively "pure" examples of Modern Denominational Yoga include later (post-1976) Transcendental Meditation and the International Society for Krishna Consciousness. Modern Denominational Yoga systems, according to de Michelis, have not had much influence in the formation of "mainstream" forms of modern yoga (de Michelis 2004: 189). In my attempt to avoid reifying these types of yoga, since they have been heterogeneous with regard to many variables, I prefer the term *modern soteriological yoga*, named for their emphasis on salvation from ordinary life.

16. The concept of stress as both a psychological and physiological syndrome is itself a modern one, having entered the vocabularies of numerous languages only since the 1930s. Hans Selye produced the earliest scholarly work (1956) on stress and argued that it is associated with urban life (see Selye 1978 [1956]). More recently, Allan Young demonstrates that stress continues to be associated with urban life (Young 1980: 134). Stress is notorious for lacking a single definition (for a discussion on the ways people have defined stress, see King, Stanley, and Burrows 1987). For a critical essay on the discourse on stress, see Young 1980.

17. I discussed Muktananda as a yoga entrepreneur first in "Branding Yoga: The Cases of Iyengar Yoga, Siddha Yoga, and Anusara Yoga" (Jain 2012a) and then in "Muktananda: Entrepreneurial Godman, Tantric Hero" (Jain 2014b). In

Chapter Four, I will return to the topics of Muktananda and Siddha Yoga in an attempt to elucidate how Siddha Yoga functions as a "yoga brand" and to explore the brand's demise as a consequence of scandals surrounding Muktananda.

18. On this tantric variety of hatha yoga, see Chapter One.

19. Peter Brent includes an account of Muktananda as godman prior to his first world tour (Brent 1972: 230–282).

20. Since Brent's visit to the ashram, the Trust has added an open-air pavilion capable of holding hundreds of people at a time, additional housing, classrooms, large auditoriums, and several dining facilities.

21. The current Siddha Yoga guru, Chidvilasananda, makes shaktipat and Siddha Yoga celebrations available to thousands at a time by means of webcasts.

22. Publicly, Muktananda held himself to standards beyond that of ordinary individuals. He suggested, for example: "The Guru should possess every virtue...He cannot be a true Guru if he engages in business, in different material pursuits or therapies...or if he indulges in sense pleasures. A disciple who discovers such behavior in a guru can only benefit by considering him a worm of bad conduct and rejecting him" (Muktananda 1985: 10). In another context, he asserted: "Just as we expect a disciple to be high and ideal, we should expect a Guru to be high and ideal. The Guru should have the power to cause an inner awakening in his disciple. He should be well versed in all the scriptures, he should be able...to transmit knowledge directly. He should have extraordinary skill in instructing his disciples. This is what a true Guru is like" (Muktananda 1994: 371).

23. Swami Durgananda describes the consequences of such organizational developments: "The birth of SYDA Foundation marked a major organizational shift from a system in which most ashram decisions were referred directly to Swami Muktananda, to a departmental system with regulated channels of communication. The Siddha Yoga centers, which had to date been independent and as idiosyncratic as each individual who ran them, also fell under the governance of SYDA Foundation, which began now to set up standards, structures, and systems of accountability for the dissemination of teachings" (Durgananda 1997: 95).

24. My first discussion of preksha dhyana as a Terapanth Jain attempt to join the competitive global yoga market appeared as "The Intersection of *Preksha* and Late Capitalism: Consumer Culture, Commodity Exchange, and the Sacred" (Jain 2010b). A later discussion appeared as "The Dual-Ideal of the Ascetic and Healthy Body: The Jain Terāpanth and Modern Yoga in the Context of Late Capitalism" (Jain 2012b).

25. Terapanth monastics wear the mouth-shield to prevent the undesired inhalation and consequent destruction of organisms in the air.

26. There are three meanings attributed to the name of this sect (*panth*) based on the multiple meanings of *tera* in Rajasthani. According to legend, *Terapanth*

was first applied to Bhiksu's order because he had thirteen (tera) monastic and thirteen lay followers. It may also refer to the thirteen Jain rules for ascetic discipline. Another explanation is that tera refers to "your" (Mahavira's) path (panth). Bhiksu taught that a radical distinction existed between two realms of value: the *laukika* or "worldly" and the *lokottara* or "spiritual." The worldly category consists of any action directed toward earning worldly benefits or merit, such as feeding a beggar or saving an animal from slaughter. In contrast, the spiritual category includes true religious practice oriented around ahimsa and the purification of the soul from karma, such as fasting or celibacy. Bhiksu argued that only spiritual behavior was appropriate for monastics since they aim toward release from the cycle of rebirth.

27. On attracting converts to the Jain tradition through the dissemination of preksha dhyana, see Jain (2014a).

28. This is a common expression that contemporary members of the Terapanth use to refer to the aim of the Anuvrat movement.

29. All Jains adopt these vows. However, monastics take the vows literally, whereas lay people fulfill the vows to the best of their ability as social actors, hence the status as "lesser" vows.

30. The JVB center in Ladnun eventually became the JVB Institute, which offered degrees in 1991 and was renamed JVB University in 2006. Representatives consider it "the first Jain university" (Jain Vishva Bharati University 2009). "Muni" or "silent one" is a common title for male monastics in India.

31. On premodern Jain yoga, see Chapter One. Tulsi believed that a uniquely Jain form of yoga had been central to the practice of Mahavira but was gradually lost, and he wanted Nathmal to rediscover this system by means of research on ancient Jain literature as well as personal experimentation.

32. Acharya Mahaprajna, personal communication, Ladnun, Rajasthan, June 28, 2009.

33. *Saman* is derived from the Sanskrit term *shramana*, which means "striver" and is used as a title for renouncers in India. It is used in the sense of one who "strives" for release from the cycle of rebirth.

34. The first initiation of saman in 1980 included six samanis. Today, there are over a hundred samanis. Of the four samanas initiated in 1986, only two remain samanas, while the other two have been initiated as monks. There have been no additional initiations of samanas since 1986.

35. For a study of canonical rules (*dharma*) and customary rules (*maryada*) in saman life, see Flugel 2003. Usually, saman only wear the mouth-shield while performing morning and evening prayers.

36. Contemporary Terapanth monastics often describe innovations to their tradition by the acharyas as "changing with the times."

37. According to Jain ontology, there are a plurality of selves trapped in and veiled by the material world. The Jain adherent adopts a rigorous ascetic path for the sake of unveiling his or her true self.

38. Several samanis confirmed that antaryatra is a form of kundalini yoga. Samani Vishubh Prajna, personal communications, Ladnun, Rajasthan, June 23–25, 2009. Samani Vinay Prajna and Samani Sanmati Prajna, multiple personal communications, Houston, Texas, 2006–2009.

39. I encountered this vision of yoga postures as preliminary to the meditational program in my conversations with numerous samanis and also in much of the literature published by Jain Vishva Bharati. Two samanis especially emphasized postures' preliminary role (Samani Madhur Prajna and Samani Vishubh Prajna, repeated personal communications, Ladnun, Rajasthan, June 2009).

40. Preksha dhyana is based on a hatha yogic vision of the structure of the subtle body, which is composed of *prana* (subtle energy or breath), *nadis* (subtle veins through which prana flows), and *chakras* (concentrated points or "wheels" of prana). The *sushumna* is the central nadi that runs along the spinal column and is surrounded by two additional nadis. *Ida* is located on the left side of the spinal column and *pingala* is on the right. The flow of prana in these two nadis must be in balance in order for prana to properly flow through the sushumna. This metaphysical understanding of the subtle body is coupled with a physiological one. Mahaprajna gives explicit physiological function to the subtle body when he argues that ida is also responsible for activating the parasympathetic system, whereas pingala activates the sympathetic system (Mahaprajna 2000: 16). To achieve a state of health, such physiological systems must be in balance.

41. Samanis and lay Terapanth scholars at JVB University want to organize scientific studies to test the physiological effects of preksha dhyana. They hypothesize that such tests will prove its effectiveness for improving health (Samani Malli Prajna, personal communication, Ladnun, Rajasthan, June 28, 2009). Mahaprajna and the samanis often refer to yoga as "physiotherapy."

42. Samani Madhur Prajna, repeated personal communications, Ladnun, Rajasthan, June 2009; Samani Vinay Prajna, repeated personal communications, Houston, Texas, 2006–2009; and Samani Rohit Prajna, London, the United Kingdom, personal communication, July 25, 2009.

43. Samani Sanmati Prajna, repeated personal communications, Houston, Texas, 2006–2009; and Samani Rohit Prajna, personal communication, London, the United Kingdom, July 25, 2009.

44. Samani Sanmati Prajna, personal communication, Houston, Texas, October 20, 2006.

45. In London, in fact, no members of the Terapanth and very few Jains come to yoga classes. Almost all of those in attendance are self-identifying Hindus. Samani Prasanna Prajna and Samani Rohit Prajna, personal communications, London, the United Kingdom, July 25, 2009.

46. Samani Madhur Prajna and Samani Vishubh Prajna, multiple personal communications, Ladnun, Rajasthan, June 2009.

47. For example, a samani once told me about an event that occurred while some samanis were traveling by car across India. Tulsi was acharya at the time. They found themselves on a narrow road (not uncharacteristic of India's rural areas) with a deep ditch on either side. Suddenly, a large truck appeared on the road coming from the opposite direction at a fast speed, and the samanis were certain that their driver would not be able to avoid a head-on collision. They closed their eyes and prayed to Tulsi, offering themselves in devotion to him. When they opened their eyes, they were on the other side of the truck, as if their car had been miraculously lifted up, carried over the truck, and placed back down safely onto the road. They attributed this event to the miraculous intervention of their guru.

48. Although Terapanth *munis* (monks) and *sadhvis* (nuns) must consistently move from one place to another except during the *chaturmas*, the monsoon season, Mahaprajna permanently settled in Ladnun in his old age. In June 2009, he turned ninety years old, thus initiating a large influx of devotee visitors. In the Terapanth, monks and nuns are allowed to settle down permanently if their health or age prevents them from being able to travel long distances by foot.

49. Personal communications, Jaipur, Rajasthan, July 2009.

50. I do not believe, however, that the JVB centers will replace other Jain centers in the diaspora communities in which they are found, since many diaspora Jains do not associate with the samanis, whom they consider "not really Jain" because they are concerned with yoga and meditation. I have heard this several times through personal communications with Jains attending the one other nonsectarian Jain center in Houston, Texas, the Jain Society of Houston.

51. I witnessed both announcements as they were made at Mahaprajna's public ninetieth birthday celebration at the JVB University in Ladnun, Rajasthan, June 22, 2009.

52. On the ethnic and religious metanarratives of Maharishi and Prabhupada, see the following articles: on Maharishi, see Humes 2005; on Prabhupada, see Goswami and Gupta 2005.

53. Bhagwan Shree Rajneesh (known in his later life as Osho), on the other hand, publicly prescribed otherwise esoteric dimensions of tantra by marketing his "neo-tantrism" to Americans and Europeans in the 1970s and 1980s. His neo-tantrism simultaneously promised absolute freedom, instant deification, physical indulgence, and sensual pleasure (Urban 2003: 241).

54. For more on Muktananda's improprieties, see Chapter Four.

55. Strauss cites Fuchs 1990.

56. Chidananda became president of the Divine Life Society in 1963 after Sivananda's death.

CHAPTER 4

1. Earlier discussions of John Friend and Anusara Yoga as a yoga brand appeared as Jain 2012a and Jain 2012d.

2. The Wanderlust Festival is a large-scale music and yoga festival (see Wanderlust 2011).

3. Friend set this precedent as early as 1998 when he officially located himself and Anusara Yoga in the Siddha Yoga lineage with the following epigraph to the *Anusara Yoga Teacher Training Manual*: "This manual on teaching hatha yoga is lovingly offered at the lotus feet of my yoga teacher, Gurumayi Chidvilasananda, who taught me the most important element of teaching yoga—divine love" (Friend 2009).

4. Dawn Dobni and George M. Zinkhan suggest, although the definition of *brand image* is not stable, there is consensus concerning four essential elements of the concept: "brand image is the concept of a brand that is held by the consumer"; "brand image is largely a subjective and perceptual phenomenon that is formed through consumer interpretation, whether reasoned or emotional"; "brand image is not inherent in the technical, functional or physical concerns of the product. Rather, it is affected and molded by marketing activities, by context variables, and by the characteristics of the perceiver"; and "where brand image is concerned, the perception of reality is more important than the reality itself" (Dobni and Zinkhan 1990: 118).

5. I am drawing from C. Whan Park, Bernard J. Jaworski, and Deborah J. MacInnis' normative framework of brand concept management consisting of a sequential process of selecting, introducing, elaborating, and fortifying a brand concept, which guides the brand image over time (Park, Jaworski, and MacInnis 1986: 135–145).

6. Many recent articles in popular yoga publications, such as *Yoga Journal*, evidence that contemporary practitioners of postural yoga colloquially often self-identify as *yogis*. As mentioned in Chapter One, in South Asian premodern yoga traditions, the term was not in use until the twelfth- to thirteenth-century emergence of the Nath Yogi tradition. According to David Gordon White, "The Nath Yogīs were and remain the sole South Asian order to self-identify as yogis" (White 2012: 17).

7. The greater the setup costs, the less likely consumers are to move to another, even better, ware, especially when such a move requires additional costs (Zauberman 2003: 405–419).

8. I discussed Siddha Yoga as a yoga brand and Muktananda as a yoga entrepreneur first in Jain 2012a and again in Jain 2014b.

9. Sarah Caldwell suggests that Muktananda's selective strategy is analogous to what David Gordon White calls the "dissembling strategy" of Abhinavagupta, the medieval Kashmiri Shaiva responsible for reconstructing the Kula tradition.

Abhinavagupta relegated the transgressive dimensions of the Kula tradition to secrecy in order to win over the "hearts and minds of the general Kashmiri populace" (see White 1999: 255; Caldwell 2001: 25).

10. Theoretically, Siddha Yoga was democratic in these ways, but, beginning in 1974, initiates had to pay for admission to an Intensive where they would receive shaktipat, thus making shaktipat inaccessible to those who could not afford the price of admission.

11. The following excerpt from one of Muktananda's published books succinctly captures the guru's general attitude about the democratic nature of Siddha Yoga: "Our time is different from the orthodox era when certain people were prohibited from studying the scriptures...recently, the sage Dayananda broke the bonds of the orthodox attitude toward women and people of lower caste...It is obvious that the orthodox restrictions are not applied in Siddha Yoga Dham; everyone chants the *Rudram*, which is a portion of the *Rig Veda*. Everyone should read and understand the scriptures. By performing good actions, a person should make himself a pure temple of God and worship the Lord of the Self within" (Muktananda 1985: 189).

12. As mentioned in note 11, initiates have to pay for admission to an Intensive where they receive shaktipat, thus making shaktipat inaccessible to those who cannot afford the price of admission. Nevertheless, as mentioned in Chapter Three, making shaktipat readily accessible to a global audience made Siddha Yoga unique because of shaktipat's historical rarity and relative unavailability (Muller-Ortega 1997: 410).

13. Further solidifying his ties to Siddha Yoga, Friend accepted an invitation from Chidvilasananda to join the Siddha Yoga Professors and Scholars Department. Through his involvement in that department, Friend befriended many scholars of Siddha Yoga, including Douglas Renfrew Brooks, Paul Muller-Ortega, William Mahony, and Sally Kempton (then Swami Durgananda), thus forming a network that would continue to influence his thinking about and dissemination of yoga (Williamson 2014: 216). These scholars would eventually collaborate on the edited volume, *Meditation Revolution*, which offers a history and theology of Siddha Yoga (1997). In August 2004, Friend taught his last yoga program at the Siddha Yoga ashram, after which Chidvilasananda closed the ashram to visitors (Williamson 2014: 225).

14. The accusations were reposted by blogger Yoga Dork in early February from an anonymous site.

CHAPTER 5

1. I first discussed regulatory attempts in Texas in Jain 2011d.

2. On the TWC, see State of Texas 2011d. On the Texas Education Code, see State of Texas 2011c.

3. Similar professional yoga associations exist in other parts of the world, including the Berufsverband der Yogalehrenden (BDY) in Germany, the Yoga Federation of Iran, and Yoga Alliance U.K.

4. On the TYA's response to regulatory attempts, see Texas Yoga Association 2011.

5. Some opponents of the popularization of postural yoga, however, do describe yoga as "religious" and as essentially Hindu. We will discuss in detail definitions of yoga as Hindu in Chapter Six, but suffice it to say here that some popular evangelical Christian leaders have proclaimed that Christians should not practice yoga because it is Hindu, and some fundamentalist Hindus agree that yoga is indeed Hindu and has been illegitimately coopted by members of other religions.

6. For more on Brown and his Abhyasa Yoga Center, see Abhyasa Yoga Center 2013.

7. Twentieth-century scholarship on religion witnessed a dramatic broadening of the definition of *religion*. As described by John Corrigan, "In the process, the way religion was defined was greatly enlarged, particularly during the mid-twentieth century, when the influential Protestant theologian Paul Tillich began to refer to religion as a person's 'ultimate concern,' and semiosis—a concern for signs and symbols—became a standard part of the study of religion, a project increasingly undertaken as a form of cryptanalysis, or code breaking. The reconceptualization of religion that ensued was played out in the second half of the twentieth century as theory-driven academic propensity for outing covert or cryptoreligious phenomena, so that researchers discovered in persons' exercise routines and patriotism structural features coincident with those found in world religions" (Corrigan 2004: 4).

8. This use of *sacred* comes from Émile Durkheim in his famous *The Elementary Forms of Religious Life* (2001 [1912]). See Chapter One, n. 2.

9. Certain insights into any given body of practice are generally not available to insiders, since they are conditioned to read their practice through the lens of the ideas and values on which the practice is built. Yet certain insights are also generally not available to outsiders, since they stand outside of the ideas, rituals, and values of the body of practice. Scholars take different positions on how to resolve this dilemma, which they often refer to as the *insider-outsider problem*. Russell McCutcheon (2001), on the one hand, suggests that scholars should be "critics, not caretakers"—that is, they are not responsible for considering insider perspectives. Wendy Doniger, on the other hand, argues for models that incorporate both insider and outsider perspectives. Doniger is a mythologist and thus studies myth, which one must enter (inside) to understand, although one can step outside and critically reflect back on it (see, e.g., Doniger O'Flaherty 1986 and 1998).

10. This trivialization of body-focused religious aims betrays a Protestant bias against the body that has been at work throughout the history of the modern study of religions.

11. Urban cites Jameson 1991. Marxist scholars in Europe first used the category *late capitalism* in the 1930s. Scholars in the Frankfurt School (a school of neo-Marxist critical theory and social thought associated with the Institute for Social Research at the University of Frankfurt am Main) used the term in the 1960s to refer to a late phase of capitalism, implying that capitalism would soon end. The term referred to an historical period that began after World War II and witnessed sudden economic growth. In 1972, Ernest Mandel popularized it, arguing that it features the emergence of multinational corporations, global markets, and mass consumption. American cultural theorist Fredric Jameson used *late capitalism* as a category for the cultural critique of what he considered postmodernity. Urban also uses it as a category for cultural critique.

12. Albanese suggests that it would be too simplistic to equate the new forms of yoga that began to emerge in the nineteenth century with tantra. However, as a comparative category, tantra provides a useful lens for understanding a certain metaphysical compatibility of both the New Age movement and postural yoga with the context of consumer culture.

13. Hanegraaff cites C. J. Bleeker's notion of religion as that which provides answers and prescriptions for dealing with human weakness and suffering with the promise of "salvation" (Hanegraaff 1998: 44; Hanegraaff cites Bleeker 1958: 127–128).

14. Samani Sanmati Prajna, personal communication, Houston, Texas, October 20, 2006.

15. Three of the four JVB centers run by samanis outside of India are in the United States; according to a 2012 study, of those practicing yoga in the United States, 82.2 percent are women and 17.8 percent are men (Macy 2012). In line with these statistics, far more women have attended preksha dhyana postural yoga classes since the 1980s when the samanis began teaching outside of India. Furthermore, in January 2009 Mahaprajna officially announced that the samanis are no longer allowed to teach male students because of the samanis' potential role as objects of the sexual desire of such students (Samani Akshay Prajna and Samani Vinay Prajna, personal communication, Houston, Texas, April 17, 2009). Other samanis, through personal communications, have emphasized that it is not appropriate for them to stand in the sometimes "immodest" yoga postures in front of men.

16. Many postural yogis acknowledge that a desire for a sexier physique often leads people to yoga, but the benefits far outweigh and sometimes cause one to forget the goal of improving sex appeal (see, e.g., Isaacs 2013). As one reader points out in the comments to the article, however, "It's ironic that this article appears in a magazine (YJ) that features so many gorgeous models in their issues. Even the person in the picture that accompanies this article seems to be a model. Why?"

17. On rites of passage, see van Gennep 1965 [1908].

18. On ritual liminality, see Turner, Victor 2008 [1969].

19. According to Clifford Geertz, myths function to represent a culture's sense of proper moral behavior and feeling as well as its sense of how the world works (Geertz 1977 [1965]). In other words, myths provide models for moral behavior as well as models of reality.

20. Singleton points out that there is nothing in the verses that Jois cites that pertains in any way to either the sequence or its individual postures (Singleton 2010: 221–222, n. 4).

21. My first discussion of the sacred and ethical (or nonethical) dimensions of Sai Baba appeared in Jain 2011a. I discussed the topic again in Jain 2011b.

22. I first discussed the ethical (or nonethical) status of yoga and other Indian mystical traditions in Jain and Kripal 2009. See also Schweitzer 1977: 9–10, 79–81; Nelson 1998; Gier 2000; Kripal 2002.

23. Although Tennant acknowledges a religious dimension of her yoga discipline, she criticizes "hard-core yogis" for which yoga functions as a "religious ritual" (Tennant 2005). Interestingly, this captures a Protestant hostility toward overt ritual practice.

24. The Holy Yoga website (2007–2010b) notes that classes will soon be available not only throughout the United States, but also in Japan, the Philippines, Germany, the United Kingdom, Mexico, India, Afghanistan, and Africa.

25. For a detailed discussion of contemporary Christian opposition to yoga because of its perceived Hindu essence and consequent conflict with Christianity, see Chapter Six.

26. Choudhury is responsible for constructing the yoga brand Bikram Yoga. Its products and services are some of the most widely purchased yoga commodities in the yoga market today. In September 2011, Choudhury filed an infringement suit against Gumucio for coopting Bikram Yoga's postural techniques. In June 2012, the United States Copyright Office decided that, since yoga proponents claim that yoga improves health, yoga postures are not eligible for copyright. For more on Choudhury's attempts to copyright certain postural yoga components, see the Conclusion.

27. The first purpose-made yoga mat was manufactured and sold by Hugger Mugger in the 1990s (Brooks, Janet Rae 2003).

28. Of course, that explanation, which had to include critical analysis of postural yoga as a body of practice in order to offer something new, ultimately had to privilege the outsider perspective. But I sought to critically analyze postural yoga while seriously considering insider perspectives in service to an adequate explanation.

CHAPTER 6

1. My first response to this movement appeared as "Is Downward Dog the Path to Hell?" (Jain 2010a). I responded again in a short essay, "The Malleability of

Yoga: A Response to Christian and Hindu Opponents of the Popularization of Yoga" (2012c) and then in an article, "Who Is to Say Modern Yoga Practitioners Have It All Wrong? On Hindu Origins and Yogaphobia" (Jain 2014c).

2. Scholarly debate over the question of whether yoga is, in fact, Hindu is not new, as was evidenced by the several papers that addressed this question at the 2011 Annual Meeting of the American Academy of Religion. The Hinduism Group hosted a panel called "Yoga Debates: Old and New." Most notable for the current chapter, Frederick M. Smith's paper discussed the interplay between the Patanjala Yoga of the *Yoga Sutras*, Vedanta, and South Asian local practices, suggesting that locally constituted yoga traditions were distinct from textual traditions (Smith, Frederick 2011). Mark Singleton's paper pointed out that nineteenth- and twentieth-century transnational constructions of postural yoga are modern reformulations of yoga (Singleton 2011). The North American Hindu Association of Dharma Studies hosted the "Is Yoga Hindu?" panel. Most notable, Edwin Bryant argued that yoga cannot be said to be Hindu even from the perspective of the *Yoga Sutras*, since that tradition requires the practitioner to move beyond identifications of the self with notions tied to the mind–body complex, which includes religious identity. He added that the *Bhagavad Gita* traditions state that individuals outside of the Brahmanic fold, and therefore outside of what is traditionally categorized as Hindu, can attain the highest states of *bhakti* or "devotion" (Bryant 2011). Christopher Key Chapple suggested that the South Asian yoga traditions betray philosophical underpinnings of pluralism and so cannot be limited by a Hindu definition (Chapple 2011). And finally, at the Society for Hindu-Christian Studies panel on "Yoga and Christianity," I argued that the historical malleability of yoga suggests that yoga cannot accurately be described as essentially Hindu (Jain 2011e).

3. This is premised on a narrow vision of religion that defines it in terms of belief. That vision has been privileged among Protestants and Catholics since the seventeenth century (Smith, Wilfred Cantwell 1991 [1962]). The implication is that a person cannot rationally adopt two religions at the same time because that would entail commitment to two different, and incompatible, belief systems.

4. Christian opponents of the popularization of yoga are not limited to the United States. Warnings against Christians' embrace of yoga occur beyond the American context, including, for example, in Ireland and the United Kingdom.

5. Many contemporary postural yogis assume that their discipline can be traced to a single South Asian lineage going back thousands of years. In Chapter Four, for example, I suggested that one important way that Iyengar elaborated the Iyengar Yoga brand was by associating it with the yoga of the *Yoga Sutras*. Yet contemporary postural yogis represent a variety of yoga systems that cannot be reduced to a set of essential characteristics, and that variety is represented in popular yoga publications, such as *Yoga Journal*, and in umbrella organizations and conferences, such as Yoga Alliance. Even the most popular postural yoga

systems today, most significantly Bikram Yoga, Iyengar Yoga, and Vinyasa, represent different brands that vary dramatically with regard to what their products and services entail and what they signify for consumers. Furthermore, there is no direct transmission between the South Asian premodern yoga traditions and modern postural yoga (Singleton 2010: 29–33). Although the modern association between yoga and health is in part a result of premodern ideas about yoga, those ideas do not survive in contemporary postural yoga (Alter 2005: 120).

6. On *fundamentalism*, see Chapter Two, n. 2.

7. Said defines Orientalism as "a system of representations framed by a whole set of forces that brought the Orient into Western learning, Western consciousness, and later, Western empire...a product of certain political forces and activities" (Said 1978: 202–203). In the colonial period, Orientalist scholarship served to legitimate colonial rule by bifurcating the world into the *Orient* and the *Occident*. The Orient and the Occident were defined in terms of perceived essences, and thus each was perceived as a homogenous, static system. Because Orientalist thinkers have defined the Orient vis-à-vis the Occident, the system of representation Said calls Orientalism reveals more about Occidental subjectivity than about any reality underlying representations of the Orient.

8. Although this chapter focuses on popular discourse, the critical study of yoga is also threatened by essentialist definitions of yoga. Scholars since the nineteenth century have largely neglected or demeaned tantra and certain narrative and practical yoga traditions because of biases in favor of analytical texts, especially the *Yoga Sutras*, and against what were perceived as degenerate religious forms, such as tantra (see Brooks, Douglas Renfrew 1990: 209, n. 8; Samuel 2008: 15–16; and White 2009: xii–xiii). In Chapter Five, we saw that some contemporary scholars, including Georg Feuerstein, Jeremy Carrette, and Richard King, betray similar biases. Postural yoga is sometimes treated as a mere accretion or commodification that distracts from the purity of the true or original yoga tradition (Feuerstein 2003; Carrette and King 2005). More recently, Loriliai Biernacki stated that the recent debate over the origins and ownership of yoga raised issues about many Hindu concepts that have become a part of American culture, including karma and meditation, and argued, "All of these ideas are Hindu in origin, and they are spreading. But they are doing it in a way that leaves behind the proper name, the box that classifies them as 'Hinduism'" (Vitello 2010). Sarah Strauss has defined yoga in limited Hindu terms, as simply a broad philosophical perspective (*yoga-darsana*) normally considered one of the six *darsanas* of Hinduism (Strauss 2005: 3).

9. Gottschalk and Greenberg define Islamophobia as such: "'Islamophobia' accurately reflects a *social* anxiety toward Islam and Muslim cultures that is largely unexamined by, yet deeply ingrained in, Americans...[T]his phobia results for most from distant social experiences that mainstream American culture

has perpetuated in popular memory, which are in turn buttressed by a similar understanding of current events…This anxiety relies on a sense of otherness, despite many common sources of thought" (Gottschalk and Greenberg 2007: 5).

10. Although I focus on Christian opposition to the popularization of yoga here, Christians are not the only opponents; some Muslims oppose it as well. Just as there is no fixed Christian position on yoga, there is no fixed Islamic position. Some Muslims, however, have suggested that yoga practice of any kind is not compatible with an authentic Muslim life because yoga is essentially Hindu. In some Muslim-majority countries, including Malaysia, Egypt, Singapore, and Indonesia, Muslim clerics have reacted to the popularization of yoga by issuing fatwas against it, declaring it *haram* or forbidden by Islamic law. Even in the cosmopolitan and diverse culture of New York City, some Muslims have reacted negatively to their fellow Muslims embracing yoga (Nir 2012).

11. Affiliated with The Christian and Missionary Alliance, Nyack College (initially named the Missionary Training Institute) was the first Bible college in North America. It was established in 1882 in New York City. In 1897 the school moved to the former location of Bernard's Clarkstown Country Club in the village of South Nyack, New York. In 1956 the school was renamed Nyack Missionary College, and again it was renamed to Nyack College in 1972.

12. As discussed in Chapter Five, some contemporary Christians argue instead that the universal psychological and physical benefits of yoga can be separated from the Hindu, Buddhist, Jain, or other doctrine-specific expressions and then reconstructed as a component of the Christian life.

13. According to *Kyria*, "Jan Brown is a freelance writer, apologist, and ministry consultant." She has also written on the incompatibility of Mormonism and evangelical Christianity (Brown, Jan 2008: 46). *Kyria* was a Christian digital magazine and website for women. It was published by *Christianity Today*, which also publishes the print magazine, *Today's Christian Woman*. In August 2012, *Kyria* merged into *Today's Christian Woman*, which is now a digital magazine and website as well as a print magazine.

14. Robaina wrote this article in response to Agnieszka Tennant's article, "Yes to Yoga" (Tennant 2005), discussed in Chapter Five.

15. The Christian Coalition of America is an evangelical Christian organization that is politically influential on both national and local levels (see Christian Coalition of America 2013).

16. De Michelis refers to Vivekananda's book *Raja Yoga* (1896) as the "seminal text" of "Modern Yoga" (de Michelis 2004: 3). In that text, Vivekananda prescribes a narrow vision of *raja yoga*. Vivekananda uses the term to refer only to what he considers authentic yoga according to his neo-vedantic, selective reading of the *Yoga Sutras*. (See discussion of Vivekananda in Chapter Two.)

17. Mohler ominously begins this article (2004) with an epigraph from Carol Midgley's article in *The Times of London*: "In the beginning there was the Church. And people liked to dress up in their best clothes and go there on Sundays and they praised the Lord and it was good. But it came to pass that people grew tired of the Church and they stopped going, and began to be uplifted by new things such as yoga and t'ai chi instead. And, lo, a spiritual revolution was born" (Midgley 2004: 4–5).

18. On "smears that Obama is neither a genuine Christian nor a genuine American," see, e.g., Posner 2010.

19. As discussed in Chapter Two, Vivekananda made a largely negative assessment of hatha yoga: "[Hatha yoga] deals entirely with the physical body, its aim being to make the physical body very strong. We have nothing to do with it here, because its practices are very difficult and cannot be learnt in a day, and, after all, do not lead to much spiritual growth. Many of these practices— such as placing the body in different postures—you will find in the teachings of Delsarte and others. The object in these is physical, not spiritual...The result of hatha-yoga is simply to make men live long; health is the chief idea, the one goal of the hatha-yogi" (Vivekananda 1982 [1896]: 23; on Delsarte, the nineteenth-century French creator of a form of gymnastics based on coordination of voice, breath, and body that became popular in areas of Europe and the United States and influenced the construction of postural yoga, see Singleton 2010: 144). Singleton argues, "Vivekananda makes an emphatic distinction between the *merely physical* exercises of *hatha* yoga, and the *spiritual* ones of 'raja yoga,' a dichotomy that obtains in modern yoga up to the present day" (Singleton 2010: 71; on Vivekananda's elision of yoga's physical elements, see de Michelis 2004: 149–180; Singleton 2010: 70–75; Jain 2011c).

20. It is ironic that the popularization of postural yoga was, in part, possible because of the missionary work of Vivekananda, a figure who opposed the physical techniques that are central to postural yoga, since he familiarized many Americans, Europeans, and Indians with the idea that yoga could be "universally" beneficial.

21. In 2002, there was a transnational public outcry in response to Choudhury and the BYCI's attempts to enforce copyrights. For more on the controversy surrounding Choudhury and the BYCI, see the Conclusion.

22. The Government of India's definition of yoga is also inclusive of various traditions, not excluding postural yoga, and simultaneously locates its origins in the ancient Indian text, Patanjali's *Yoga Sutras*: "Yoga is one of the six systems of Vedic philosophy. Maharishi Patanjali, rightly called 'The Father of Yoga,' compiled and refined various aspects of Yoga systematically in his 'Yoga Sutras' (aphorisms). He advocated the eight folds path of Yoga, popularly known as 'Ashtanga Yoga,' for all-round development of human beings. They are: Yama, Niyama, Asana, Pranayama, Pratyahara, Dharana, Dhyana and Samadhi. These

components advocate certain restraints and observances, physical discipline, breath regulations, restraining the sense organs, contemplation, meditation and samadhi. These steps are believed to have a potential for improvement of physical health by enhancing circulation of oxygenated blood in the body, retraining the sense organs thereby inducing tranquility and serenity of mind. The practice of Yoga prevents psychosomatic disorders and improves an individual's resistance and ability to endure stressful situations" (Department of AYUSH 2010).

23. On scholarly debates over yoga's claimed origins in the Indus Valley Civilization, see Chapter One.

24. For example, Mohler is the current President of the Southern Baptist Theological Seminary, and A. Shukla is a co-founder of the HAF and currently sits on its Board of Directors.

25. Said makes the same argument in his 1994 Afterword to *Orientalism*: "[C]ultures are hybrid and heterogenous and...cultures and civilizations are so interrelated and interdependent as to beggar any unitary or simply delineated description of their individuality" (Said 1994: 347). Many contemporary scholars of yoga, discussed in Chapter One, make a similar argument for culturally and historically situated visions of yoga.

26. Andrew J. Nicholson (2010) suggests that, although nineteenth-century thinkers constructed the unifying notion of Hinduism, a unified Hindu identity has South Asian roots in fourteenth- to seventeenth-century Vedantic philosophers who unified the Vedanta, Samkhya, and Yoga philosophical schools, as well as the devotional traditions focused on Shiva, Vishnu, and Shakti under a single umbrella by envisioning them as separate streams leading to a single ultimate reality, Brahman. These South Asian philosophers influenced later nineteenth-century Hindu reformers and, in turn, Orientalist thinkers.

27. Examples of this type of Orientalist scholarship include H. H. Wilson's *Essays and Lectures, Chiefly on the Religion of the Hindus* (1828) and Monier Monier-William's *Hinduism* (1894).

28. Reform movements, including the Brahmo Samaj, the Arya Samaj, and the Ramakrishna Mission (founded by Vivekananda), sought to correct the gap between rationalist Hinduism, which was perceived to restore a great and pure Hinduism of the ancient past, and corrupt, ritualistic Hinduism. Contemporary Hindu nationalist organizations continue to reify such a binary, including the contemporary Rashtriya Svayam Sevak Sangh (RSS), the Vishva Hindu Parishad (VHP), and the Bharatiya Janata Party (BJP), which seek to unite Indian Hindus against what are perceived as foreign powers and influences (on nineteenth-century and contemporary reform and nationalist movements, see Flood 1996: 250–265). Attempts by some contemporary Hindus to rigidly define Hindu religious identity have served to justify hostilities between communities and political positions (see, e.g., the essays in Ludden 2006). Samuel argues, however, "the societies of South Asia before, say, the

mid-nineteenth-century, while not entirely free from religious conflicts, had much more fluid and less categorical conceptualizations of religious identity than we now see" (Samuel 2008: 14).

29. The Hindu reformist and Orientalist attempts to identify a set of canonical Hindu analytical texts reflect their tendency to privilege a Protestant "template" for religion, which defines it categorically in terms of what are perceived as original and authentic texts (Samuel 2008: 15–16). Much of this excludes South Asian folk and popular religious ideas, narratives, and practices that have existed alongside Buddhist, Jain, Hindu, and Islamic ideas and practices (Brooks, Douglas Renfrew 1990: 209, n. 8; White 2009: xii–xiii). These include religious elements, such as polytheism, ritual, devotion, tantra, and yoga's body practices, that are deemed inferior to so-called rational elements. On the category of tantra, which traditionally includes hatha yoga, Douglas Renfrew Brooks points out that, until recently, it was neglected as a serious object of study and was instead treated as "an unwanted stepchild in the family of Hindu studies" because of the "residual historical prejudice" of those "influenced by the christocentric attitudes that marked nineteenth-century Sanskrit scholarship" (Brooks, Douglas Renfrew 1990: 209, n. 8).

30. The edited volume *Invading the Sacred: An Analysis of Hinduism Studies in America* provides a substantive selection of the arguments waged against American scholarship on Indian religions (Ramaswamy, de Nicolas, and Banerjee 2007).

31. Strategies that reify a Hindu definition of yoga are premised on the idea that yoga has its "origins" in Hinduism. For example, Groothuis argues that proponents of yoga base their teachings on the "ancient Hindu" Vedas, which serve as the "primary scriptures of Hinduism" (Groothuis 2010), and the HAF maintains that yoga dates back over five thousand years to the Indus Valley Civilization (HAF 2009b). This argument assumes that the Indus Valley Civilization represents an early form of Hinduism, an issue that is debated based on the perceived cultural interaction between the Indus Valley Civilization and Indo-Europeans (see Chapter One, n. 6). On the scholarly debate over whether or not archaeological artifacts from the Indus Valley civilization provide evidence of yoga, also see Chapter One.

32. In Chapter One, I discussed the need to consider the diversity of yoga and the exchanges involved in its history. In short, an argument for an exclusively Hindu definition of yoga is problematic, since the history of yoga suggests that there was a "general climate of thought" in which participants drew from and reworked a shared set of religio-philosophical categories as well as textual traditions (Samuel 2008: 216). Examples include exchanges between the Buddhist Madhyamika school (second century c.e.), the Buddhist Yogacara school (third to fourth century c.e.), schools based on the *Yoga Sutras* (fourth to fifth century c.e.), Advaita Vedanta (circa eighth century c.e.), and Haribhadra Yakini-Putra's Jain *Yoga Drishti Samuccaya* (eighth century c.e.) (on exchanges between traditions, see, e.g., De la Vallée Poussin 1936–1937; Dixit 1968; Larson 1989; Bronkhorst 1993; Bronkhorst 1998; Chapple 2003; Qvarnström 2003: 131–133;

Samuel 2008: 216–218, 232). For these reasons, Samuel suggests we take *yoga* "in a wide sense" that includes the variety of closely entwined Buddhist, Jain, Hindu, and other practices (2007: 179).

33. Because, for Groothuis, yoga is about an experience of oneness with Brahman, he argues that it is a "depersonalizing, deindividualizing, dehumanizing practice" (Groothuis 2010). Although this argument could be made for certain premodern yoga traditions—those, for example, that require the practitioner to "disintegrate" subjectivity (see Grinshpon 2002)—it is not true for all yoga traditions. As discussed in Chapter Five, for example, although the "liminal space" of the postural yoga class is a space set apart from everyday life (de Michelis 2004; see also Chapter Five), it does not require the practitioner to "disintegrate" subjectivity. Rather, postural yoga functions as a time for the practitioner to undergo psychological and physical healing and transformation through reducing stress and improving physical fitness.

34. In Chapter One, I discussed several of the various methods and aims of premodern yoga systems. According to the *Yoga Sutras*, for example, the key method for attaining release from suffering is meditation whereby one realizes the self as pure consciousness, distinct from the mind–body complex (Larson 2012). This is, however, not the only aim of yoga discussed in the *Yoga Sutras* (see White 2006: 10). The *Bhagavad Gita* suggests that the key method for attaining release from suffering is concentration on "the one and only highest self, the god Kṛṣṇa" (Malinar 2012: 58). In the Nath yoga tradition, on the other hand, hatha yoga methods are used for the transmutation of the subtle and physical bodies in order to acquire bodily immortality, sexual pleasure, as well as supernatural and sociopolitical powers (White 1996; White 2009). As discussed in preceding chapters, although postural yoga shares with premodern yoga an emphasis on training and controlling the mind–body complex, it has been repurposed for the sake of modern conceptions of health, beauty, and self-development (Alter 2004; de Michelis 2004; Strauss 2005; Newcombe 2007; Singleton 2010). Furthermore, as discussed in Chapter Five, the "liminal space" of the postural yoga class is a space set apart from the stresses of everyday life (de Michelis 2004; see n. 1), but it does not represent a renunciation of everyday life as is found in some premodern yoga systems.

35. As discussed in Chapters One and Two, prior to the twentieth century, posture practice was not central to any yoga tradition (see de Michelis 2004; Alter 2005; Singleton 2010). Hatha yoga, which developed as an adjunct to the Nath yoga tradition's practices, did involve a variety of postures but only in preparation for "internal sexual practices"—that is, the tantric manipulation of the subtle body (Samuel 2008: 279, 336). In nineteenth-century India, the tantric manipulation of the subtle body began to be elided from popular yoga practice because of the negative view of tantra and hatha yoga among Orientalist scholars and Hindu reformers (Singleton 2010: 41–80). Unsurprisingly, the yoga systems

that underwent the greatest degree of popularization were those postural varieties that elided tantric elements completely, such as Iyengar Yoga, Ashtanga, and
Bikram Yoga. Hatha yoga is the traditional source of postural yoga. For example, British teacher of postural yoga and co-founder of YogaLondon Rebecca
French suggests that what most people in the West think of as yoga is *hatha*
yoga, which French describes as a path towards enlightenment that focuses on
building physical and mental strength (Kremer 2013). Yet, equating postural
yoga and hatha yoga does not account for the historical sources, which include
British military calisthenics (Sjoman 1996), modern medicine (Alter 2004), and
the physical culture of European gymnasts, bodybuilders, martial experts, and
contortionists (Singleton 2010). All of these influenced figures responsible for
constructing postural yoga, including Krishnamacharya and, in turn, his three
most influential students—Iyengar, K. Pattabhi Jois, and T. K. V. Desikachar—
who shaped popularized forms of postural yoga (Singleton 2010). Such an equation would also fail to account for the variety of methods and aims that hatha
yoga systems themselves have embraced since their emergence in the tenth to
eleventh centuries that are usually not present in postural yoga (see n. 34).

36. Urban points out that whereas "Indian mysticism was imagined as some-
    thing otherworldly and identified with Vedānta or other philosophical
    schools…Tantra represented, for both Indian and European authors, mysti-
    cism in its most degenerate form: a kind of mysticism that had been corrupted
    with sensual desire and this-worldly power" (Urban 2003: 15, n. 53). Because
    the "degenerate" vision of tantra included yoga's body practices, those prac-
    tices were also disdained in the early history of modern yoga (de Michelis
    2004; Singleton 2010) and continue to be disdained by representatives of the
    Christian yogaphobic position and the Hindu origins position.

37. Although there are Hindu vestiges in many postural yoga contexts—con-
    sider the names of certain postures, such as the *nataraja asana*, named for a
    famous image of the Hindu deity Shiva as "Lord of the Dance," or the invo-
    cation to Patanjali at the beginning of many Iyengar Yoga classes—these do
    not point to the survival of premodern soteriological methods and aims of
    yoga. Their presence is explained by Singleton's argument that nineteenth-
    and twentieth-century constructors of postural yoga wanted to prescribe
    this form of fitness as something that was indigenous to India (Singleton
    2010) and by my suggestion in Chapter Four that efforts to tie certain yoga
    brands to an ancient lineage served to elaborate those brands. Furthermore,
    the aims of postural yoga do not reflect the soteriological systems of premod-
    ern Hindu traditions, including the use of the body as a means to a nondual-
    ist enlightenment experience as found in many tantric traditions. Rather,
    postural yoga's aims include modern conceptions of self-development.

38. Rather than establish an American religion, the U.S. Constitution protects reli-
    gious freedom, meaning it frees individuals to choose and practice religions

independent of the state, therefore protecting religions from the state and the state from any single, majority religion. Since many of the founders of the United States were deeply religious deists and free thinkers who themselves held minority religious viewpoints, the separation of religions and the state for the sake of protecting against persecution of religious minorities is not surprising.

39. The Hindu origins position evidences Singleton's argument that Vivekananda's dichotomy between the "mere" physical yoga of hatha yoga and the spiritual yoga of raja yoga "obtains in modern yoga up to the present day" (Singleton 2010: 71). Scholars, however, agree that this dichotomy is based on a mistaken historical understanding. White (2006) argues against the vision of yoga, based largely on Vivekananda's selective reading of the *Yoga Sutras*, as an inner-directed practice, based on a "closed" model of the body, and points out that yoga is often about the body as "open" (White 2006: 6–12).

40. Groothuis (2010), on the other hand, conflates postural yoga with the yoga of Vivekananda even though Vivekananda boldly disavowed those body techniques and aims that became central to postural yoga (see n. 16).

CONCLUSION

1. For a more detailed discussion of this case, see Chapter Six.

2. Fish cites the two federal court cases involving the BYCI: first, *Bikram Choudhury v. Kim Schreiber-Morrison, Mark Morrison, and Prana Incorporated*, case No. SA02-565 DOC(ANX) (USDC Central District of CA, Southern Division); and second, *Open Source Yoga Unity v. Bikram Choudhury*, case No. C 03-03182 PJH (USDC Northern District of CA, San Francisco Division). She points out that, despite settlements out of court, the two cases took almost three years to resolve, from 2002 to 2005 (Fish 2006: 203, n. 31).

3. The Copyright Office decided "a claim in a compilation of exercises or the selection and arrangement of yoga poses will be refused registration" (Office of the Federal Register 2012: 37607).

4. For the details of this case, I primarily rely on Ernst 2003: 205–206.

5. Jonathan Z. Smith (1990) suggests that much scholarship on comparing religions was influenced by competing Protestant and Catholic claims regarding the center or essence of "true Christianity."

6. King borrows Ludwig Wittgenstein's *family resemblance* approach to defining religions. Wittgenstein suggests that no religion is defined by merely a central or essential quality; rather, religions, like families, are defined insofar as they share a series of delimited qualities (Wittgenstein 1953).

7. On the polythetic approach, Doniger cites Wittgenstein on his concept of family resemblance (see Wittgenstein 1953). On other scholars of religion who apply the polythetic approach to Hinduism, Doniger cites Brian K. Smith (1987) and Axel Michaels (2004 [1998]).

Bibliography

Abhyasa Yoga Center. 2013. http://www.abhyasayogacenter.com/essays/profession. html.

Africa Yoga Project. 2014. "About Africa Yoga Project." Accessed April 5, 2014. http://www.africayogaproject.org/pages/about-us.

Albanese, Catherine L. 2007. *A Republic of Mind and Spirit: A Cultural History of American Metaphysical Religion*. New Haven, CT: Yale University Press.

———. 2012. *America: Religions and Religion*. 5th ed. Belmont, CA: Wadsworth Publishing.

Alter, Joseph S. 1994. "Celibacy, Sexuality, and the Transformation of Gender into Nationalism in North India." *Journal of Asian Studies* 53(1) (February): 45–66.

———. 2004. *Yoga in Modern India: The Body Between Science and Philosophy*. Princeton, NJ: Princeton University Press.

———. 2005. "Modern Medical Yoga: Struggling with a History of Magic, Alchemy and Sex." *Asian Medicine, Tradition and Modernity* 1(1): 119–146.

Alvarez, Lizette. 2010. "Bending With a Holy Twist." *New York Times*, November 27. Accessed May 1, 2011. http://cityroom.blogs.nytimes.com/2010/11/27/stretching-and-bending-with-a-holy-twist/?pagemode=print.

American Marketing Association. 2012. "Resource Library." *Marketing Power*. Accessed February 5, 2012. http://www.marketingpower.com/_layouts/Dictionary. aspx?dLetter=B.

Anand, Utkarsh. 2013. "Supreme Court to Examine if Yoga can be Compulsory in Schools. *The Indian Express*, October 19. Accessed October 25. http://archive. indianexpress.com/news/supreme-court-to-examine-if-yoga-can-be-compulsory-in-schools/1184494/.

Anusara, Inc. 2009a. "About Anusara Philosophy." *Anusara: Yoga, Shri, Community*. Accessed March 7, 2012. http://www.anusara.com/index.php?option=com_cont ent&view=article&id=51&Itemid=85.

———. 2009b. "Books." *Anusara: Yoga, Shri, Community*. Accessed March 7, 2012. http://www.anusara.com/index.php?option=com_virtuemart&Itemid=143.

———. 2009c. "Ethical Guidelines." *Anusara: Yoga, Shri, Community*. Accessed March 7, 2012. http://www.anusara.com/index.php?option=com_content&view=article &id=71&Itemid=188.

——. 2009d. "Online Store." *Anusara: Yoga, Shri, Community.* Accessed March 7, 2012. http://www.anusara.com/index.php?option=com_virtuemart&Itemid=53.

Appadurai, Arjun. 1999. "Globalization and the Research Imagination." *International Social Science Journal* 51(160): 229–238.

Arnould, Eric J., and Craig J. Thompson. 2005. "Consumer Culture Theory (CCT): Twenty Years of Research." *Journal of Consumer Research* 31 (March): 868–869.

Asad, Talal. 1993. *Genealogies of Religion: Discipline and Reasons of Power in Christianity and Islam.* Baltimore, MD: The Johns Hopkins University Press.

Author unknown. 1909a. "Yoga Divides Theosophy Ranks." *Chicago Daily Tribune,* September 19: 3.

Author unknown. 1909b. "Yoga Followers Shut Out of Hall." *Chicago Daily Tribune,* September 20: 8.

Author unknown. 1911a. "The Heathen Invasion of America." *Current Literature* 51(5) (November): 538.

Author unknown. 1911b. "A Hindu Apple for Modern Eve." *Los Angeles Times,* October 22: III, 20.

Author unknown. 1911c. "This Soul Destroying Poison of the East: The Tragic Flood of Broken Homes and Hearts, Disgrace and Suicide That Follows the Broadening Stream of Morbidly Alluring Oriental 'Philosophies' into Our Country." *Washington Post,* May 28.

Author unknown. 1941. "Speaking of Pictures…This is Real Yoga." *Time,* February 24.

Babb, Lawrence A. 1987. *Redemptive Encounters: Three Modern Styles in the Hindu Tradition.* New Delhi: Oxford University Press.

Baker, Deborah. 2008. *A Blue Hand: The Beats In India.* New York: Penguin Press.

Baudrillard, Jean. 2002. *Jean Baudrillard: Selected Writings.* 2nd ed., edited by Mark Poster. Translated by Jacques Mourrain. Stanford, CA: Stanford University Press.

Bellah, Robert N., Richard Madsen, William M. Sullivan, and Steven M. Tipton. 2007 [1985]. *Habits of the Heart: Individualism and Commitment in American Life.* 3rd ed. Los Angeles: University of California Press.

Berger, Peter. 1979. *The Heretical Imperative: Contemporary Possibilities of Religious Affirmation.* New York: Doubleday.

Bharati, Agehananda. 1976. *The Light at the Center: Context and Pretext of Modern Mysticism.* Santa Barbara, CA: Ross-Erikson.

Billard, Mary. 2010a. "A Yoga Manifesto." *New York Times,* April 23. Accessed April 23, 2010. http://www.nytimes.com/2010/04/25/fashion/25yoga.html?ref=homepage &src=me&pagewanted=print.

——. 2010b."Their Lotus Can't Take Root on a Yoga Mat." *New York Times,* October 1. Accessed October 1, 2010. http://www.nytimes.com/2010/10/03/fashion/03noticed. html?_r=1&emc=eta1&pagewanted=print.

Birney, Bernadette. 2012. "My Resignation Letter." *Bernadette Birney.* Accessed March 7, 2012. http://bernadettebirney.com/2012/02/my-resignation-letter.html.

Black, Brian. 2007. "Eavesdropping on the Epic: Female Listeners in the *Mahābhārata*." In *Gender and Narrative in the Mahābhārata*, edited by Simon Brodbeck and Brian Black, 53–78. New York: Routledge.

Blavatsky, Helena P. 1888. *The Secret Doctrine*. Vol. 1. Theosophical University Press Online Edition. Accessed November 1, 2010. www.theosociety.org/pasadena/sd/sd1-1-05.htm.

Bleeker, C. J. 1958. *Godsdienst Voorheen en Thans: Beschouwingen over de Structuur van het Geloof*. Servire: Den Haag.

Bocock, Robert. 1993. *Consumption*. New York: Routledge.

Bouy, Christian. 1994. *Les Nātha Yogin et Les Upaniṣads, Étude d'histoire de la littérature Hindoue*. Collège de France, Publications de l'Institut de Civilisation Indienne. Paris: Édition-Diffusion de Bocard.

Brent, Peter. 1972. *Godmen of India*. New York: Quadrangle Books.

Bronkhorst, Johannes. 1981. "Yoga and Seśvara Sāmkhya." *Journal of Indian Philosophy* 9: 309–320.

———. 1993. *The Two Traditions of Meditation in Ancient India*. Delhi: Motilal Banarsidass.

———. 1998. *The Two Sources of Indian Asceticism*. 2nd ed. Delhi: Motilal Banarsidass.

———. 2007. *Greater Magadha: Studies in the Culture of Early India*. Leiden, The Netherlands: Brill.

———. 2011. "The Brahmanical Contribution to Yoga." "Contextualizing the History of Yoga in Geoffrey Samuel's *The Origins of Yoga and Tantra*: A Review Symposium." *International Journal of Hindu Studies* 15(3): 303–357.

Brooks, Douglas Renfrew. 1990. *The Secret of the Three Cities: An Introduction to Hindu Śakta Tantrism*. Chicago: University of Chicago Press.

———. 1997. "The Canons of Siddha Yoga: The Body of Scripture and the Form of the Guru." In *Meditation Revolutions: A History and Theology of the Siddha Yoga Lineage*, edited by Douglas Renfrew Brooks, Swami Durgananda, Paul E. Muller-Ortega, William K. Mahony, Constantina Rhodes Bailly, and S. P. Sabharathnam, 277–346. South Fallsburg, NY: Agama Press.

Brooks, Douglas Renfrew, Swami Durgananda, Paul E. Muller-Ortega, William K. Mahony, Constantina Rhodes Bailly, and S. P. Sabharathnam, editors. 1997. *Meditation Revolutions: A History and Theology of the Siddha Yoga Lineage*. South Fallsburg, NY: Agama Press.

Brooks, Janet Rae. 2003. "Yoga-Supply House Fit for a Market; Utah-built company reflects strength of founder's vision." *Salt Lake Tribune*, May 11.

Brown, Candy Gunther. 2013. "Declaration of Candy Gunther Brown." In Motion for the Issuance of an Alternative Writ of Mandamus; Memorandum of Points and Authorities. Declaration of Jennifer Sedlock, Candy Gunther Brown, Ph.D., and Dean R. Broyles, Esq. "Resources." *The National Center for Law and Policy*. Accessed January 15, 2014. http://www.nclplaw.org/resources/.

Brown, J. 2005. "Practice as Profession." Accessed November 3, 2012. http://www.abhyasayogacenter.com/essays/profession.html.

Brown, Jan. 2001. "What You Need to Know About New Age Beliefs." *Today's Christian Woman* 23/5: 52.

———. 2008. "Understanding Mormonism." *Today's Christian Woman* 30/1: 46.

Bryant, Edwin. 2011. Comments presented at the annual meeting of the North American Hindu Association of Dharma Studies in conjunction with the annual meeting of the American Academy of Religion, San Francisco, CA, November 19–22.

Bryant, Edwin, and Maria Ekstrand. 2004. *The Hare Krishna Movement: The Postcharismatic Fate of a Religious Transplant.* New York: Columbia University Press.

Buckner, Julie. 2011. "The Wizard of Wanderlust: John Friend and the Yoga of Recognition." *AOL Healthy Living: Spirit,* August 10. Accessed March 7, 2012. http://www.huffingtonpost.com/julie-buckner/wanderlust-yoga-festival_b_922116.html?view=print&comm_ref=false.

Caldwell, Sarah. 2001. "The Heart of the Secret: A Personal and Scholarly Encounter with Shakta Tantrism in Siddha Yoga." *Nova Religio: The Journal of Alternative and Emergent Religions* 5(1) (October): 9–51.

Carrette, Jeremy, and Richard King. 2005. *Selling Spirituality: The Silent Takeover of Religion.* New York: Routledge.

Catalfo, Phil. n. d. "Is Yoga a Religion." *Yoga Journal.* Accessed May 16, 2011. http://www.yogajournal.com/lifestyle/283.

Chakrabarti, Dilip K. 2009. "Who Owns the Indian Past? The Case of the Indus Civilization." Lecture presented at India International Centre, New Delhi, 21 July.

Chappell, Vere. 2010. *Sexual Outlaw, Erotic Mystic: The Essential Ida Craddock.* San Francisco, CA: Weiser Books.

Chapple, Christopher Key. 1998. "Haribhadra's Analysis of Pātañjala and Kula Yoga in the Yogadṛṣṭisamuccaya." In *Open Boundaries: Jain Communities and Cultures in Indian History,* edited by John E. Cort, 15–30. New York: SUNY Press.

———. 2003. *Reconciling Yogas: Haribhadra's Collection of Views on Yoga.* Albany: State University of New York Press.

———. 2005. "Raja Yoga and the Guru: Gurani Anjali of Yoga Anand Ashram, Amityville, New York." In *Gurus in America,* edited by Thomas A. Forsthoefel and Cynthia Ann Humes, 15–35. New York: State University of New York Press.

———. 2008. *Yoga and the Luminous: Patañjali's Spiritual Path to Freedom.* Albany: State University of New York Press.

———. 2011. "Recovering Jainism's Contribution to Yoga Traditions." "Contextualizing the History of Yoga in Geoffrey Samuel's *The Origins of Yoga and Tantra*: A Review Symposium." *International Journal of Hindu Studies* 15(3): 323–333.

Chopra, Deepak. 2010a. "Sorry, Your Patent on Yoga has Run Out." *Washington Post,* April 23. Accessed October 25, 2010. http://newsweek.washingtonpost.com/onfaith/panelists/deepak_chopra/2010/04/sorry_your_patent_on_yoga_has_run_out.html.

——. 2010b. "Yoga Belongs to All of Us." *Washington Post*, April 28. Accessed October 25, 2010. http://newsweek.washingtonpost.com/onfaith/panelists/ deepak_chopra/2010/04/yoga_belongs_to_all_of_us.html.

Choprha, Chhogmal. n.d. *A Short History of the Terapanthi Sect of the Swetamber Jains and its Tenets*. 4th ed. Calcutta: Sri Jain Swetamber Terapanthi Sabha.

Christian Coalition of America. 2013. "Welcome to the Christian Coalition of America." Accessed February 15, 2013. www.cc.org.

Church of the Holy Trinity v. United States. 1892. 143 U.S. 457.

Congregation for the Doctrine of the Faith. 1989. "Letter to the Bishops of the Catholic Church." Accessed May 1, 2011. http://www.ewtn.com/library/CURIA/ CDFMED.HTM.

Corrigan, John. 2004. Introduction: Emotions Research and the Academic Study of Religion. In *Religion and Emotion: Approaches and Interpretations*, edited by John Corrigan, 3–32. Oxford: Oxford University Press.

Cort, John E. 1987. "Medieval Jaina Goddess Traditions." *Numen* 34(2): 235–255.

——. 2000. "Worship of Bell-Ears the Great Hero, a Jain Tantric Deity." In *Tantra in Practice*, edited by David Gordon White, 417–433. Princeton, NJ: Princeton University Press.

——. 2002. "Bhakti in the Early Jain Tradition: Understanding Devotional Religion in South Asia." *History of Religions* 42(1) (August): 59–86.

CrossFit. 2013. "What is CrossFit?" Accessed January 10, 2013. http://community. crossfit.com/what-is-crossfit.

Davidson, Ronald M. 2002. *Indian Esoteric Buddhism: A Social History of the Tantric Movement*. New York: Columbia University Press.

Déchanet, Jean Marie. 1960. *Christian Yoga*. New York: Harper & Brothers Publishers.

De la Vallée Poussin, Louis. 1936–1937. "Le Bouddhisme et le yoga de Patañjali." *Mélanges Chinois et Bouddhiques* 5: 223–242.

de Michelis, Elizabeth. 2004. *A History of Modern Yoga: Patañjali and Western Esotericism*. New York: Continuum.

Department of AYUSH. 2010. "Yoga." Ministry of Health and Family Welfare. Government of India. Accessed on July 20, 2012. http://www.indianmedicine. nic.in/searchdetail.asp?lang=1&lid=33.

Despres, Loraine. n. d. "Yoga's Bad Boy: Bikram Choudhury." *Yoga Journal*. Accessed March 10, 2013. http://www.yogajournal.com/lifestyle/328?print=1.

Dhand, Arti. 2007. "Paradigms of the Good in the *Mahābhārata*: Śuka and Sulabhā in Quagmires of Ethics." In *Gender and Narrative in the Mahābhārata*, edited by Simon Brodbeck and Brian Black, 258–278. New York: Routledge.

D Magazine. 2011. "Best of Big D." Accessed May 6, 2011. http://www3.dmagazine. com/best-of-big-d.

Dixit, K. K. 1968. *The Yogabindu of Ācārya Haribhadrasūri*. Ahmedabad: Lalbhai Dalpatbhai Bharatiya Sanskriti Vidyamandira.

Dobni, Dawn, and George M. Zinkhan. 1990. "In Search of Brand Image: A Foundation Analysis." *Advances in Consumer Research* 17.

Doniger, Wendy. 2009. *The Hindus. An Alternative History*. New York: Penguin Books.

Doniger O'Flaherty, Wendy. 1986. *Dreams, Illusion, and Other Realities*. Chicago: University of Chicago Press.

——. 1998. *The Implied Spider: Politics and Theology in Myth*. New York: Columbia University Press.

Driscoll, Mark. 2010. "Mark Driscoll on Yoga." *YouTube*, July 10. Accessed October 20, 2010. http://www.youtube.com/watch?v=BhcoBLdM8CQ.

Dundas, Paul. 1998. "Becoming Gautama: Mantra and History in Svetambara Jainism." In *Open Boundaries: Jain Communities and Cultures in Indian History*, edited by John E. Cort, 31–52. New York: State University of New York Press.

——. 2000. "The Jain Monk Jinapati Suri Gets the Better of a Nath Yogi." In *Tantra in Practice*, edited by David Gordon White, 231–238. Princeton: NJ: Princeton University Press.

Durgananda, Swami. 1997. "To See the World Full of Saints: The History of Siddha Yoga as a Contemporary Movement." In *Meditation Revolutions: A History and Theology of the Siddha Yoga Lineage*, edited by Douglas Renfrew Brooks, Swami Durgananda, Paul E. Muller-Ortega, William K. Mahony, Constantina Rhodes Bailly, and S. P. Sabharathnam, 3–6. South Fallsburg, NY: Agama Press.

Durkheim, Émile. 2001 [1912]. *The Elementary Forms of Religious Life*. Translated by Carol Cosman. Oxford: Oxford University Press.

Einstein, Mara. 2008. *Brands of Faith: Marketing Religion in a Commercial Age*. New York: Routledge Press.

Eliade, Mircea. 1963. *Myth and Reality*. Translated by William R. Trask. New York: Harper and Row.

——. 1990 [1958]. *Yoga: Immortality and Freedom*. Translated by Willard R. Trask. Princeton, NJ: Princeton University Press.

——. 1991 [1952]. *Images and Symbols*. Translated by Philip Mairet. Princeton, NJ: Princeton University Press.

——. 1996 [1949]. *Patterns in Comparative Religion*. Translated by Rosemary Sheed. Introduction by John Clifford Holt. Lincoln, NE: University of Nebraska Press.

Ernst, Carl W. 2003. *Following Muhammad: Rethinking Islam in the Contemporary World*. Chapel Hill, NC: The University of North Carolina Press.

——. 2012. "A Fourteenth-Century Persian Account of Breath Control and Meditation." In *Yoga in Practice*, edited by David Gordon White, 133–140. Princeton, NJ: Princeton University Press.

Fairservis, Walter A. 1975. *The Roots of Ancient India*. Chicago: University of Chicago Press.

Featherstone, Mike. 1991. "The Body in Consumer Culture." In *The Body: Social Process and Cultural Theory*, edited by Mike Featherstone, Mike Hepworth, and Bryan S. Turner, 170–196. London: Sage.

———. 2007. *Consumer Culture and Postmodernism*. 2nd ed. London: Sage.

Featherstone, Mike, and Scott Lash. 1995. Introduction to *Global Modernities*. London: Sage Publications.

Ferro-Luzzi, Gabriella Eichinger. 1991. "The Polythetic-Prototype Approach to Hinduism." In *Hinduism Reconsidered*, edited by Gunter D. Sontheimer and Hermann Kulke, 187–195. New Delhi: Manohar Publications.

Feuerstein, Georg. 2003. "The Lost Teachings of Yoga." *Common Ground*, March. Accessed December 1, 2011. www.commonground.ca/iss/0303140/lost_teach ings_of_yoga.shtml.

Findly, Ellison Banks. 1985. "Gārgī at the King's Court: Women and Philosophic Innovation in Ancient India." In *Women, Religion, and Social Change*, edited by Yvonne Yazbeck Haddad and Ellison Banks Findly, 37–58. Albany, NY: State University of New York Press.

Firat, A. Fuat, and Alladi Venkatesh. 1995. "Liberatory Postmodernism and the Reenchantment of Consumption." *Journal of Consumer Research* 22(3) (December): 239–267.

Fish, Allison. 2006. "The Commodification and Exchange of Knowledge in the Case of Transnational Commercial Yoga." *International Journal of Cultural Property* 13: 189–206.

Fitzgerald, James L. 2012. "A Prescription for *Yoga* and Power in the *Mahābhārata*." In *Yoga in Practice*, edited by David Gordon White, 43–57. Princeton, NJ: Princeton University Press.

Flood, Gavin. 1996. *An Introduction to Hinduism*. Cambridge: Cambridge University Press.

Flugel, Peter. 2003. "The Codes of Conduct of the Terāpanth Samaṇ Order." *South Asia Research* 23(1) (May): 7–53.

Folan, Lilias. 2013. "What is Yoga." *Thoughts from Lilias*, May 6. Accessed on May 15, 2013. http://www.liliasyoga.com/modules/blockblog/blockblog-post. php?post_id=15.

Fox. James. 2008–2010. *Prison Yoga Project*. Accessed April 5, 2014. www.prison-yoga.com

Friend, John. 2009a. *Anusara Teacher Training Manual*. 12th ed. The Woodlands, TX: Anusara Press.

———. 2009b. "John's Blog." *Anusara: Yoga, Shri, Community*, August 15. Accessed March 7, 2012. https://www.anusara.com/index.php?option=com_ wpmu&m=200908&blog_id=2&Itemid=12.

———. 2012. *John Friend, Sridaiva Yoga*. Accessed January 15, 2014. http://www.john friend.us.

Fuchs, C. 1990. *Yoga in Deutschland: Rezeption-Organisation-Typologie*. Stuttgart: Kohlhammer.

Fuller, C. J. 2004 [1992]. *The Camphor Flame: Popular Hinduism and Society in India*. Revised and expanded ed. Princeton, NJ: Princeton University Press.

Geertz. 1977 [1965]. "Religion as a Cultural System." *The Interpretation of Cultures*. New York: Basic Books.

Gelberg, Steven J. 1989. "Exploring an Alternative Reality: Spiritual Life in ISKCON." *Krishna Consciousness in the West*, edited by David G. Broomley and Larry D. Shinn. Lewisburg, PA: Bucknell University Press.

Giddens, Anthony. 1991. *Modernity and Self-Identity: Self and Society in the Late Modern Age*. Cambridge: Polity Press.

Gier, Nicholas F. 2000. *Spiritual Titanism: Indian, Chinese, and Western Perspectives*. Albany, NY: State University of New York Press.

Goldberg, Philip. 2010. *American Veda: From Emerson and the Beatles to Yoga and Meditation*. New York: Random House.

Gombrich, Richard, and Gananath Obeyesekere. 1988. *Buddhism Transformed: Religious Change in Sri Lanka*. Princeton, NJ: Princeton University Press.

Goswami, Tamal Krishna, and Ravi M. Gupta. 2005. "Krishna and Culture: What Happens When the Lord of Vrindavana Moves to New York City." In *Gurus in America*, edited by Thomas A. Forsthoefel and Cynthia Ann Humes. New York: State University of New York Press.

Gottschalk, Peter, and Gabriel Greenberg. 2007. *Islamophobia*. New York: Rowman & Littlefield Publishers.

Grinshpon, Yohanan. 2002. *Silence Unheard. Deathly Otherness in Pātañjala-Yoga*. Albany, NY: State University of New York Press.

Groothuis, Doug. 2010. "The Meaning of Yoga: A Conversation with Stephanie Syman and Doug Groothuis." "Thinking in Public," *AlbertMohler.com*, September 20. Accessed September 21, 2010. http://www.albertmohler.com/2010/09/20/the-meaning-of-yoga-a-conversation-with-stephanie-syman-and-doug-groothius/.

Halbfass, Wilhelm. 1988. *India and Europe: An Essay in Understanding*. Albany, NY: State University of New York Press.

Hanegraaff, Wouter J. 1998. *New Age Religion and Western Culture: Esotericism in the Mirror of Secular Thought*. Albany, NY: State University of New York Press.

Heelas, Paul. 1996. *The New Age Movement: The Celebration of the Self and the Sacralization of Modernity*. Cambridge, MA: Oxford University Press.

Hemacandra. 2002. *The Yogaśāstra of Hemacandra: A Twelfth-Century Handbook on Śvetāmbara Jainism*. Translated by Olle Qvarnström. Cambridge, MA: Harvard University Press.

Hiltebeitel, Alf. 1978. "The Indus Valley 'Proto-Siva', Re-examination Through Reflection on the Goddess, the Buffalo, and the Symbolism of the *vāhanas*." *Anthropos* Bd. 73 (H. 5./6.): 767–779.

Hindu American Foundation. 2009a. "Hindu Americans Take Global Stage at Parliament of World Religions." Posted on December 13, 2009. Accessed October 24, 2010. http://www.hafsite.org/media/pr/haf-prw.

———. 2009b. "Yoga Beyond Asana." Accessed on October 22, 2010. http://www. hafsite.org/media/pr/yoga-hindu-origins.

Holpuch, Amanda. 2013. "Evangelical Christian Group Helps Sue California School Over Yoga Classes." *The Guardian*, January 10. Accessed January 11, 2013. http://www.theguardian.com/world/2013/jan/10/christian-parents-sue-california-school-yoga.

Holt, Douglas B. 2002. "Why do Brands Cause Trouble? A Dialectical Theory of Consumer Culture and Branding." *Journal of Consumer Research* 29 (June): 71–72.

Holy Yoga. 2007–2010a. "Brook Boon, Founder." Accessed November 13, 2012. https://holyyoga.net/about/3/.

———. 2007–2010b. "Holy Yoga." Accessed November 13, 2012. http://holyyoga.net.

Horwell, V. 1998. "First Time Here?" The Guardian Travel. *The Guardian* (August 29): 12.

Huffstutter, P. J. 2009. "Missouri's Yoga Enthusiasts Go to the Mat Over Sales Tax." *Los Angeles Times*. Accessed November 1, 2012. http://articles.latimes. com/2009/dec/18/nation/la-na-yoga-tax18-2009dec18.

Humes, Cynthia Ann. 2005. "Maharishi Mahesh Yogi: Beyond the TM Technique." In *Gurus in America*, edited by Thomas A. Forsthoefel and Cynthia Ann Humes. New York: State University of New York Press.

Huyssen, Andreas. 1986. *After the Great Divide: Modernism, Mass Culture, Postmodernism*. Bloomington, IN: Indiana University Press.

ILEA Further and Higher Education Sub-Committee. 1968. "Report Submitted on 2 September 1968 by the Education Officer and Presented on 10 July 1968." (May/June) London Metropolitan Archives, ILEA/CL/PRE/16/17.

Inden, Ronald B. 1990. *Imagining India*. Cambridge: Blackwell.

Isaacs, Nora. n. d. "Positive I. D." *Yoga Journal*. Accessed March 10, 2013. http:// www.yogajournal.com/lifestyle/1243?print=1.

Iyengar, B. K. S. 1966. *Light on Yoga*. New York: Schocken.

———. 1988. *The Tree of Yoga: Yoga Vrksa*, edited by Daniel Rivers-Moore. San Francisco, CA: The Aquarian Press.

Jain, Andrea R. 2010a. "Is Downward Dog the Path to Hell? Evangelicals and Fundamentalist Hindus Come Together in their Denunciation of Yoga's Popularity in the U.S." *Religion Dispatches*, October 27. Accessed August 1, 2012. http://www. religiondispatches.org/archive/3616/is_downward_dog_the_path_to_hell/.

———. 2010b. "The Intersection of *Preksha* and Late Capitalism: Consumer Culture, Commodity Exchange, and the Sacred." *Health, Well-Being, and the Ascetic Ideal: Modern Yoga in the Jain Terapanth*. Doctoral dissertation. Rice University.

———. 2010c. "The Terapanth: A History." *Health, Well-Being, and the Ascetic Ideal: Modern Yoga in the Jain Terapanth*. Doctoral dissertation. Rice University.

———. 2011a. "Death of a Self-Proclaimed God-Man: Sai Baba's Controversial Career." *Religion Dispatches*, May 1. Accessed May 2, 2011. http://www.religiondispatches. org/archive/culture/4547/death_of_a_self-proclaimed_god-man%3A_sai_baba%27s_controversial_career/.

——. 2011b. "God, Man: Sai Baba and the Ethical Status of Gurus." *Himal Southasian*, June. Accessed July 1, 2011. http://www.himalmag.com/component/content/article/4495-god-man.html.

——. 2011c. "No, I Don't Owe My Yoga Mat to Vivekananda." *Religion Dispatches*, October 4. Accessed October 4, 2011. http://www.religiondispatches.org/archive/culture/5216/no%2C_i_don't_owe_my_yoga_mat_to_vivekananda.

——. 2011d. "'Soul of Yoga' at Stake in Texas Regulation Push." *Religion Dispatches*, May 18. http://www.religiondispatches.org/archive/culture/4624/'soul_of_yoga'_at_stake_in_texas_regulation_push/.

——. 2011e. "The Unlimited Meaning and Function of Yoga: A Response to Christian and Hindu Opponents of the Popularization of Yoga." Paper presented at the Society for Hindu-Christian Studies in conjunction with the annual meeting for the American Academy of Religion, San Francisco, CA, November 19–22.

——. 2012a. "Branding Yoga: The Cases of Iyengar Yoga, Siddha Yoga, and Anusara Yoga." *Approaching Religion* 2(2): 3–17.

——. 2012b. "The Dual-Ideal of the Ascetic and Healthy Body: The Jain Terāpanth and Modern Yoga in the Context of Late Capitalism." *Nova Religio* 15(3) (February): 29–50.

——. 2012c. "The Malleability of Yoga: A Response to Christian and Hindu Opponents of the Popularization of Yoga." *Journal of Hindu-Christian Studies* 25: 3–10.

——. 2012d. "Yoga Guru or CEO? Saving the Brand When Scandal Strikes." *Religion Dispatches*, March 9. Accessed March 9, 2012. http://www.religiondispatches.org/archive/culture/5716/yoga_guru_or_ceo_saving_the_brand_when_scandal_strikes.

——. 2014a. "Conversion to Jain Traditions." In *Oxford Handbook of Religious Conversions*, edited by Charles Farhadian and Lewis R. Rambo, 444–464. New York: Oxford University Press.

——. 2014b. "Muktananda: Entrepreneurial Godman, Tantric Hero." In *Gurus of Modern Yoga*, edited by Ellen Goldberg and Mark Singleton, 190–209. New York: Oxford University Press.

——. 2014c. "Who Is to Say Modern Yoga Practitioners Have It All Wrong?: On Hindu Origins and Yogaphobia." *Journal of the American Academy of Religion* 82(2) (June): 427–471.

Jain, Andrea R., and Jeffrey J. Kripal. 2009. "Quietism and Karma: Non-Action as Non-Ethics in Jain Asceticism." *Common Knowledge, Symposium: Apology for Quietism* Part 2, 15(2) (Spring): 197–207.

Jain Vishva Bharati University. 2009. Accessed April 4, 2009. http://www.jvbi.ac.in.

Jameson, Frederic. 1991. *Postmodernism: Or, the Cultural Logic of Late Capitalism*. Durham, NC: Duke University Press.

——. 1998. "Postmodernism and Consumer Society." In *The Anti-Aesthetic: Essays on Postmodern Culture*, edited by Hal Foster. New York: New Press.

Johnson, Benton. 1992. "On Founders and Followers: Some Factors in the Development of New Religious Movements." *Sociological Analysis* 53(S): S1–S13.

JVB Houston. 2007. *Newsletter*, April. Accessed August 23, 2011. http://www.jvb-houston.org/newsletters.htm.

———. 2011. "Daily Schedule." Accessed on August 23, 2011. http://www.jvbhouston.org/dailyschedule.htm.

Kakar, Sudhir. 1983. *Shamans, Mystics and Doctors: A Psychological Inquiry into India and its Healing Traditions*. Boston, MA: Beacon Press.

Kaminoff, Leslie and Amy Matthews. 2012. *Yoga Anatomy*, illustrated by Sharon Ellis. Second Edition. Champaign, IL: Human Kinetics.

Kashi Company. 2013. "Meet Us." Accessed January 17, 2013. http://www.kashi.com/meet_us.

King, Michael, Gordon Stanley, and Graham Burrows. 1987. *Stress: Theory and Practice*. Sydney: Grune and Stratton.

King, Richard. 1999. *Orientalism and Religion: Postcolonial Theory, India and "The Mystic East."* New York: Routledge.

Kremer, William. 2013. "Does Doing Yoga Make You a Hindu." *BBC*, November 20. Accessed November 21, 2013. http://www.bbc.com/news/magazine-25006926.

Kripa Foundation. 2006–2007. *Kripa Foundation*. Accessed April 5, 2014. http://www.kripafoundation.org.

Kripal, Jeffrey J. 1998. *Kali's Child: The Mystical and the Erotic in the Life and Teachings of Ramakrishna*. 2nd ed. Chicago: University of Chicago Press.

———. 2002. "Debating the Mystical as the Ethical: An Indological Map." In *Crossing Boundaries: Essays on the Ethical Status of Mysticism*, edited by G. William Barnard and Jeffrey J. Kripal, 15–69. New York: Seven Bridges Press/Chatham House.

Laidlaw, James. 1995. *Riches and Renunciation: Religion, Economy, and Society Among the Jains*. New York: Oxford University Press.

Laine, Joy. 2011. "Contemporary Yoga and its Contested Domains." Paper presented at the annual meeting for the American Academy of Religion, San Francisco, CA, November 19–22.

Larson, Gerald James. 1989. "An Old Problem Revisited: The Relation Between Sāmkhya, Yoga and Buddhism." *Studien zur Indologie und Iranistik* 15: 129–146.

———. 1999. "Classical Yoga as Neo-Sāmkhya: A Chapter in the History of Indian Philosophy. *Asiatische Studien* 53(3): 723–732.

———. 2012. "Pātanjala Yoga in Practice." In *Yoga in Practice*, edited by David Gordon White, 73–96. Princeton, NJ: Princeton University Press.

Lau, Kimberly J. 2000. *New Age Capitalism: Making Money East of Eden*. Philadelphia, PA: The University of Pennsylvania Press.

Laughing Lotus. 2012. *Laughing Lotus*. Accessed January 1. www.laughinglotus.com.

Lawrence, Stewart J. 2012. "The Anusara Yoga Scandal: Can a $6 Billion Industry Salvage Its Image?" *The Huffington Post*, February 13. Accessed March 7. http://www.huffingtonpost.com/stewart-j-lawrence/anusara-yoga-scandal_b_1272471.html.

Leviton, Richard. 1990. "From Sea to Shining Sea." *Yoga Journal* March/April: 57–65.

Lewis, Waylon. 2012. "My Interview with John Friend Regarding *jfexposed* Accusations." *Elephant Journal*, February 8. Accessed March 7. http://www.elephantjournal.com/2012/02/my-interview-with-john-friend-regarding-ijfexposedi-accusations/.

Lindquist, Steven E. 2008. "Gender at Janaka's Court: Women in the Bṛhadāraṇyaka Upaniṣad Reconsidered." *Journal of Indian Philosophy* 36(3): 405–426.

Locklin, Reid, and Julia Lauwers. 2009. "Rewriting the Sacred Geography of Advaita: Swami Chinmayananda and the Sankara-Dig-Vijaya." *Journal of Hindu Studies* 2(2): 179–128.

Love, Robert. 2010. *The Great Oom: The Improbable Birth of Yoga in America.* New York: Viking.

Ludden, David, editor. 2006. *Making India Hindu: Religion, Community, and the Politics of Democracy in India.* 2nd ed. New York: Oxford University Press.

Lyon, David. 2000. *Jesus in Disneyland: Religion in Postmodern Times.* Cambridge: Polity Press.

MacArthur, John. 2007. Interview by Erica Hill. "Prime News with Erica Hill." CNN, September 11.

Macy, Dayna. 2008. "Practitioner Spending Grows to Nearly $6 Billion a Year." Press Release for *Yoga Journal.* Accessed February 26, 2008. http://www.yoga-journal.com/advertise/press_releases/10.

———. 2012. "Yoga Journal Releases 2012 'Yoga in America' Market Study." Press Release for *Yoga Journal.* Accessed May 2, 2013. http://www.yogajournal.com/press/yoga_in_america?print=1.

Mahāprajña, Ācārya. 2000. *Prekṣadhyāna: Śarīraprekṣa.* Jīvan-Vijñan Granthmala [Science of Living Series] 7. Lāḍnūn, Rājasthān: Jain Vishva Bharati.

———. 2003a. *Prekṣadhyāna: Caitanya Kendra Prekṣa.* Jīvan-Vijñan Granthmala [Science of Living Series] 8. Lāḍnūn, Rājasthān: Jain Vishva Bharati.

———. 2003b. *Preksha Dhayana: Perception of Body,* edited by Muni Mahendra Kumar. Lāḍnūn, Rājasthān: Jain Vishva Bharati.

———. 2004. *Prekṣa Dhyāna: Theory and Practice,* edited by Muni Mahendra Kumar. Translated by Muni Mahendra Kumar and Jethalal S. Zaveri. Lāḍnūn, Rājasthān: Jain Vishva Bharati.

———. 2009 [original publication date unknown]. *Prekṣadhyāna: Siddhanta aur prayoga.* Lāḍnūn, Rājasthān: Jain Vishva Bharati.

Main, Darren. 2011. *The Yogi Entrepreneur: A Guide to Earning a Mindful Living Through Yoga.* San Francisco, California: Surya House Publishing.

Malinar, Angelika. 2012. "Yoga Practices in the *Bhagavadgītā*." In *Yoga in Practice,* edited by David Gordon White, 58–72. Princeton, NJ: Princeton University Press.

Mallinson, James. 2005. "Rāmānandī Tyāgīs and Haṭhayoga." *Journal of Vaishnava Studies* 14(1) (Fall): 107–121.

———. 2007. *The Khecarīvidyā of Ādinātha*. A critical edition and annotated translation of an early text of hathayoga. London: Routledge.

Marcus, George E. 1995. "Ethnography in/of the World System: The Emergence of Multi-sited Ethnography." *Annual Review of Anthropology* 24(October): 95–117.

Marshall, Sir John. 1931. *Mohenjodaro and the Indus Civilization: Being an Official Account of Archaeological Excavations at Mohenjodaro Carried Out by the Government of India Between the Years* 1922–27. Volume 1. Delhi: Indological Book House.

Marty, Martin E., and R. Scott Appleby, eds. 1993–2004. *The Fundamentalism Project*. 6 vols. Chicago: University of Chicago Press.

McCutcheon, Russell T. 2001. *Critics not Caretakers: Redescribing the Public Study of Religion*. New York: State University of New York Press.

McEvilley, Thomas. 1981. "An Archaeology of Yoga." *RES: Anthropology and Aesthetics* 1 (Spring): 44–77.

Mehta, Silva, Mera Mehta, and Shyam Mehta. 1990. *Yoga: The Iyengar Way*. New York: Knopf.

Michaels, Axel. 2004. *Hinduism: Past and Present*. Princeton, NJ: Princeton University Press.

Midgley, Carol. 2004. "Spirited Away: Why the End is Nigh for Religion." *Times of London*, November 4.

Mohler, Albert. 2004. "The Re-paganization of the West: A Glimpse of the Future." AlbertMohler.com Blog, November 5. Accessed October 21, 2010. http://www.albertmohler.com/2004/11/05/the-re-paganization-of-the-west-a-glimpse-of-the-future/.

———. 2008. "The Empty Promise of Meditation." AlbertMohler.com Blog, November 20. Accessed October 25, 2010. http://www.albertmohler.com/2008/11/20/the-empty-promise-of-meditation/.

———. 2009. "Are We a Nation of Hindus?" AlbertMohler.com Blog, August 26. Accessed October 22, 2010. http://www.albertmohler.com/2009/08/26/are-we-a-nation-of-hindus/.

———. 2010a. "Help from Hindu Quarters—The New York Times on 'Take Back Yoga,'" AlbertMohler.com Blog, November 29. Accessed November 30, 2010. http://www.albertmohler.com/2010/11/29/help-from-hindu-quarters-the-new-york-times-on-take-back-yoga/.

———. 2010b. "The Meaning of Yoga: A Conversation with Stephanie Syman and Doug Groothuis." "Thinking in Public," AlbertMohler.com, September 20. Accessed September 21, 2010. http://www.albertmohler.com/2010/09/20/the-meaning-of-yoga-a-conversation-with-stephanie-syman and-doug-groothius/.

———. 2010c. "The Subtle Body—Should Christians Practice Yoga?" AlbertMohler.com Blog, September 20. Accessed on September 21, 2010. http://www.albertmohler.com/2010/09/20/the-subtle-body-should-christians-practice-yoga/.

Monier-Williams, Monier. 1894. *Hinduism*. London: Society for Promoting Christian Knowledge.

Mukhya-Niyojika, Sadhvi Vishrutavibha. 2007. *An Introduction to Terapanth*. Lāḍnūn, Rājasthān: Jain Vishva Bharati.

Muktananda, Swami. 1985. *The Perfect Relationship: The Guru and the Disciple*. South Fallsburg, NY: SYDA Foundation.

———. 1994. *Light on the Path*. South Fallsburg, NY: SYDA Foundation.

Muller, Max. 1899. *The Six Systems of Philosophy*. London: Longmans, Green.

———. 1974 [1898]. *Ramakrishna: His Life and Sayings*. With a Review of the Book by Swami Vivekananda. Calcutta: S. Gupta.

Muller-Ortega, Paul E. 1997. "Shaktipat: The Initiatory Descent of Power." In *Meditation Revolutions: A History and Theology of the Siddha Yoga Lineage*, edited by Douglas Renfrew Brooks, Swami Durgananda, Paul E. Muller-Ortega, William K. Mahony, Constantina Rhodes Bailly, and S. P. Sabharathnam, 407–444. South Fallsburg, NY: Agama Press.

Nelson, Lance E. 1998. "The Dualism of Nondualism: Advaita Vedanta and the Irrelevance of Nature." In *Purifying the Earthly Body of God: Religion and Ecology in Hindu India*, edited by Lance E. Nelson, 61–88. Albany, NY: State University of New York Press.

Newcombe, Suzanne. 2007. "Stretching for Health and Well-Being: Yoga and Women in Britain, 1960–1980." *Asian Medicine: Tradition and Modernity* 3(1): 37–63.

Nir, Sarah Maslin. 2012. "Seeking to Clear a Path Between Yoga and Islam." *The New York Times*, April 8. Accessed April 15, 2012. http://www.nytimes.com/2012/04/09/ nyregion/in-queens-seeking-to-clear-a-path-between-yoga-and-islam .html?pagewanted=all&_r=0.

Olivelle, Patrick. 1993. *The Āśrama System: History and Hermeneutics of a Religious Institution*. New York: Oxford University Press.

Otto, Rudolf. 1958 [1917]. *The Idea of the Holy: An Inquiry into the Non-rational Factor in the Idea of the Divine and its Relation to the Rational*. Oxford: Oxford University Press.

Park, C. Whan, Bernard J. Jaworski, and Deborah J. Maclnnis. 1986. "Strategic Brand Concept-Image Management." *Journal of Marketing* 50(4) (October): 135–145.

Patton, Laurie L. 2011. "Thinking Anthropologically About the History of Indian Religions." "Contextualizing the History of Yoga in Geoffrey Samuel's *The Origins of Yoga and Tantra*: A Review Symposium." *International Journal of Hindu Studies* 15(3): 312–317.

Paulist Office for Ecumenical and Interfaith Relations. n. d. "Books/DVDs." Accessed February 3, 2013. http://www.tomryancsp.org/books.htm.

PBS. 2008. "Yoga." *The Story of India*. Accessed December 2, 2012. http://www.pbs. org/thestoryofindia/gallery/photos/16.html#yoga.

Pechilis, Karen, ed. 2004. *The Graceful Guru: Hindu Female Gurus in India and the United States*. New York: Oxford University Press.

Pennington, Brian K. 2005. *Was Hinduism Invented? Britons, Indians, and the Colonial Construction of Religion*. New York: Oxford University Press.

Pew Forum. 2008. "Many Americans Say Other Faiths Can Lead to Eternal Life: Most Christians Say Non-Christian Faiths Can Lead to Salvation." "Beliefs and Practices" (December 18). Accessed October 22, 2010. http://pewforum. org/Many-Americans-Say-Other-Faiths-Can-Lead-to-Eternal-Life.aspx.

Porterfield, Amanda. 2001. *The Transformation of American Religion: The Story of a Late-Twentieth-Century Awakening*. Oxford: Oxford University Press.

Posner, Sarah. 2010. "Obama's Supposed 'Religion Dilemma' and American Exceptionalism." *Religion Dispatches*, November 19. Accessed November 20, 2010. http://www.religiondispatches.org/dispatches/sarahposner/3760/obama's_ supposed_"religion_dilemma"_and_american_exceptionalism_.

PraiseMoves. 2010. *PraiseMoves*. Accessed October 25, 2010. http://praisemoves. com/.

Qvarnström, Olle. 1998. "Stability and Adaptability: A Jain Strategy for Survival and Growth." *Indo-Iranian Journal* 41: 33–55.

——. 2000. "Jain Tantra: Divinatory and Meditative Practices in the Twelfth-Century *Yogaśāstra* of Hemacandra." In *Tantra in Practice*, edited by David Gordon White, 595–604. Princeton: NJ: Princeton University Press.

——. 2003. "Losing One's Mind and Becoming Enlightened: Some Remarks on the Concept of Yoga in Śvetāmbara Jainism and its Relation to the Nāth Siddha Tradition." In *Yoga, The Indian Tradition*, edited by Ian Whicher and David Carpenter, 130–142. London: RoutledgeCurzon.

Raj, Selva J. 2005. "Passage to America: Ammachi on American Soil." In *Gurus in America*, edited by Thomas A. Forsthoefel and Cynthia Ann Humes, 123–146. New York: State University of New York Press.

Ramamani Iyengar Memorial Yoga Institute. 2009a. "Institutions." *B. K. S. Iyengar: The Official Website*. Accessed September 5, 2012. http://www.bksiyengar.com/modules/Institut/institut.htm.

——. 2009b. "Invocation to Sage Patanjali." *B. K. S. Iyengar: The Official Website*. Accessed September 5, 2012. http://www.bksiyengar.com/modules/IYoga/sage .htm.

——. 2009c. "Teachers." *B. K.S. Iyengar: The Official Website*. Accessed September 5, 2012. http://www.bksiyengar.com/modules/Teacher/teacher.asp.

Ramaswamy, Krishnan, Antonio de Nicolas, and Aditi Banerjee. Eds. 2007. *Invading the Sacred: An Analysis of Hinduism Studies in America*. New Delhi: Rupa Publications.

Rao, Ramesh. 2010. "It is Wrong to Deny Yoga's Hindu Origins." *Guardian*, December 2. Accessed on July 1, 2011. http://www.guardian.co.uk/commentis-free/belief/2010/dec/02/yoga-hindu-rebranded-wrongly/print.

Robaina, Holly Vicente. 2005. "The Truth About Yoga." *Today's Christian Woman* 27/2: 40.

——. 2007. "Take a Pass on Yoga." *Today's Christian Woman*, January 17. Accessed June 18, 2014. http://www.todayschristianwoman.com/articles/2005/march/truth-about-yoga.html.

Robertson, Pat. 1995. *The End of the Age*. Nashville, TN: W Publishing Group.

——. 2007. *The 700 Club*. ABC, November 28.

Roof, Wade Clark. 1993. *A Generation of Seekers: The Spiritual Journey of the Baby Boom Generation*. New York: HarperCollins.

——. 1999. *Spiritual Marketplace: Baby Boomers and the Remaking of American Religion*. Princeton, NJ: Princeton University Press.

Roof, Wade Clark, and William McKinney. 1987. *American Mainline Religion: Its Changing Shape and Future*. New Brunswick, NJ: Rutgers University Press.

Rüping, Klaus. 1977. "Zur Askese in indischen Religionen." *Zeitschrift für Missionswissenschaft und Religionswissenschaft* 2: 81–98.

Russell, Cheryl. 1993. *The Master Trend: How the Baby Boom Generation is Remaking America*. New York: Plenum Press.

Said, Edward W. 1978. *Orientalism*. New York: Vintage Books.

——. 1994. *Culture and Imperialism*. New York: Vintage Books.

——. 1995. "Afterword." *Orientalism*. 25th anniversary ed. New York: Vintage Books.

——. 2004. *Humanism and Democratic Criticism*. Columbia Themes in Philosophy. New York: Columbia University Press.

Saliba, John A. 1989. "Christian and Jewish Religious Responses to the Hare Krishna Movement in the West." In *Krishna Consciousness in the West*, edited by David G. Broomley and Larry D. Shinn, 219–237. Lewisburg, PA: Bucknell University Press.

Samuel, Geoffrey. 2007. "Endpiece." *Asian Medicine: Tradition and Modernity* 3(1): 177–188.

——. 2008. *Origins of Yoga and Tantra: Indic Religions to the Thirteenth Century*. Cambridge: Cambridge University Press.

——. 2011. "Response." "Contextualizing the History of Yoga in Geoffrey Samuel's *The Origins of Yoga and Tantra*: A Review Symposium." *International Journal of Hindu Studies* 15(3): 338–350.

Schleiermacher, Friedrich. 1999 [1830]. *The Christian Faith*. Foreword by B. A. Gerrish. New York: T&T Clark Ltd.

Schmidt, Leigh Eric. 2010. *Heaven's Bride: The Unprintable Life of Ida C. Craddock, American Mystic, Scholar, Sexologist, Martyr, and Madwoman*. New York: Basic Books.

Schweitzer, Albert. 1977. *Indian Thought and Its Development*. Translated by Charles E. B. Russell. Gloucester, MA: Peter Smith.

Selye, Hans. 1978. *The Stress of Life*. 2nd ed. New York: McGraw-Hill.

Shah, Sheetal. 2010. "Yoga: It's Not About Ownership, It's About Origins." *Treehugger*, December 7. Accessed on July 1, 2011. http://www.treehugger.

com/files/2010/12/yoga-its-not-about-ownership-its-about-origins-hin du-american-foundation.php.

Shee, Monika. 1986. *Tapas und Tapasvin in den erzählenden Partien des Mahābhārata*. Reinbek: Dr. Inge Wezler Verlag.

Shellnutt, Kate. 2011. "Practicing Yoga, Practicing Faith?" *Houston Chronicle*, February 25: F6–F7.

Shri K. Pattabhi Jois Ashtanga Yoga Institute. 2009. "The Practice." Accessed March 2, 2011. http://kpjayi.org/the-practice.

Shukla, Aseem. 2010a. "Dr. Chopra: Honor Thy Heritage." *Newsweek*, April 2. Accessed on July 2, 2011. http://newsweek.washingtonpost.com/onfaith/panelists/aseem_shukla/2010/04/dr_chopra_honor_thy_heritage.html.

———. 2010b. "Hinduism and Sanatana Dharma: One and the Same." *Washington Post*, April 30. Accessed on July 2, 2011. http://newsweek.washingtonpost.com/onfaith/panelists/aseem_shukla/2010/04/hinduism_and_sanatana_dharma_one_and_the_same.html.

———. 2010c. "The Theft of Yoga." *Newsweek*, April 18. Accessed October 26, 2010. http://newsweek.washingtonpost.com/onfaith/panelists/aseem_shukla/2010/04/nearly_twenty_million_people_in.html.

Shukla, Aseem, and Sheetal Shah. 2011. "The Rape of Yoga." *The Pioneer*, June 21. Accessed on July 1, 2011. http://www.dailypioneer.com/252823/The-rape-of-Yoga.html.

Shukla, Suhag A. 2010. "Letter to Yoga Journal," Hindu American Foundation. Accessed October 24, 2010. http://www.hafsite.org/sites/default/files/YogaJournalLetter.pdf.

———. 2011. "The Origins and Ownership of Yoga." *Huffington Post*, December 3. Accessed July 1, 2011. http://www.huffingtonpost.com/suhag-a-shukla-esq/the-origins-and-ownership_b_791129.html?view=print.

Silk, Jonathan A. 1997. "Further Remarks on the *yogācāra bhikṣu*." In *Dharmadūta: Mélanges offers au Vénérable Thích Huyên-Vi á l'occasion de son soixante-dixiéme anniversaire*, edited by Bhikkhu Pāsādika and Bhikkhu Tampalawela Dhammaratana, 233–250. Paris: Éditions You Feng.

———. 2000. "The Yogācāra Bhikṣu." In *Wisdom, Compassion, and the Search for Understanding: The Buddhist Studies Legacy of Gadjin M. Nagao*, edited by Johnathan A. Silk, 265–314. Honolulu, HI: The University of Hawaii Press.

Singleton, Mark. 2010. *Yoga Body: The Origins of Modern Posture Practice*. New York: Oxford University Press.

———. 2011. "Ownership, Lineage, and the Yoga Free Market: Tracing Modern Yoga's Cultural Politics." Paper presented at the annual meeting for the American Academy of Religion, San Francisco, CA, November 19–22.

Sinha, Kounteya. 2011. "India Pulls the Plug on Yoga as Business." *The Times of India*, February 6. Accessed July 2, 2011. http://articles.timesofindia.indiatimes.com/2011-02-06/india/28355602_1_hot-yoga-patanjali-tkdl.

Sjoman, N. E. 1996. *The Yoga Tradition of the Mysore Palace*. New Delhi: Abhinav Publications.

Smith, Brian K. 1987. "Exorcising the Transcendent: Strategies for Defining Hinduism and Religion." *History of Religions* 27(1) (August): 32–55.

Smith, David. 2003. "Orientalism and Hinduism." In *Blackwell Companion to Hinduism,* edited by Gavin Flood, 45–63. Oxford: Wiley-Blackwell.

Smith, Frederick. 2011. "Religion in Search of a Philosophy: A Brief History of the Goals of Yoga." Paper presented at the annual meeting for the American Academy of Religion, San Francisco, CA, November 19–22.

Smith, Jonathan Z. 1990. *Drudgery Divine: On the Comparison of Early Christianities and the Religions of Late Antiquity.* Chicago: University of Chicago Press.

———. 1993 [1978]. *Map is Not Territory: Studies in the History of Religions.* Chicago: University of Chicago Press.

Smith, Wilfred Cantwell. 1991 [1962]. *The Meaning and End of Religion.* Minneapolis, MN: Fortress Press.

Sprockhoff, Joachim Friedrich. 1976. *Saṃnyāsa: Quellenstudien zur Askese im Hinduismus.* Volume One of Two: *Untersuchungen über die Saṃnyāsa-Upaniṣads.* Wiesbaden: Franz Steiner.

Squires, Nick. 2011. "'Harry Potter and Yoga are Evil,' says Catholic Church Exorcist." *The Telegraph,* November 25. Accessed on November 26, 2011. http://www. telegraph.co.uk/culture/harry-potter/8915691/Harry-Potter-and-yoga-are-evil-says-Catholic-Church-exorcist.html.

Srinivas, Krishna Ravi. 2007. "Intellectual Property Rights and Traditional Knowledge: The Case of Yoga." *Economic and Political Weekly* 42(27/28) (July 14–20): 2866–2867, 2869–2871.

Srinivasan, Doris. 1984. "Unhinging Siva from the Indus Civilization." *Journal of the Royal Asiatic Society of Great Britain and Ireland* 1: 77–89.

Stark, Rodney. 1996. "Why Religious Movements Succeed or Fail: A Revised General Model." *Journal of Contemporary Religion* 11: 133–146.

State of Texas. 2011a. "History: HB 1839." *Texas Legislature Online.* Accessed on May 16, 2011. http://www.capitol.state.tx.us/BillLookup/history.aspx?LegSess=82R&Bill=HB1839.

———. 2011b. "History: SB 1176." *Texas Legislature Online.* Accessed May 16, 2011. http://www.capitol.state.tx.us/BillLookup/text.aspx?LegSess=82R&Bill=SB1176.

———. 2011c. "Texas Education Code." *Texas Education Agency.* Accessed May 16, 2011. http://portals.tea.state.tx.us/page.aspx?id=920&bc=506.

———. 2011d. "Texas Workforce Commission." *Texas Workforce Commission.* Accessed May 16, 2011. http://www.twc.state.tx.us.

Storey, John. 2009. *Cultural Theory and Popular Culture: An Introduction.* 5th ed. New York: Pearson.

Strauss, Sarah. 2005. *Positioning Yoga: Balancing Acts Across Cultures.* New York: Berg.

Swallow, Deborah A. 1982. "Ashes and Powers: Myth, Rite and Miracle in an Indian God-man's Cult." *Modern Asian Studies* 16: 123–158.

Swartz, Mimi. 2010. "The Yoga Mogul." *New York Times*, July 21. Accessed March 7, 2012. http://www.nytimes.com/2010/07/25/magazine/25Yoga-t.html?pagewanted=print.

Swope, Pastor. 2008. "The Specters of Oom." *The Paranormal Pastor,* July 1. Accessed June 1, 2011. http://theparanormalpastor.blogspot.com/2008/07/specters-of-oom.html.

SYDA Foundation. 2012. "Centers." *Siddha Yoga.* Accessed May 1, 2012. http://www.siddhayoga.org/centerslist.

Syman, Stephanie. 2010. *The Subtle Body: The Story of Yoga in America.* New York: Farrar, Straus and Giroux.

Taylor, Kathleen. 2001. *Sir John Woodroffe, Tantra and Bengal: 'An Indian Soul in a European Body?'* New York: Routledge.

Tennant, Agnieszka. 2005. "Yes to Yoga: Can a Christian Breathe Air that has been Offered to Idols?" *Christianity Today* 49. Accessed October 25, 2010. http://www.christianitytoday.com/ct/2005/mayweb-only/42.0b.html.

Texas Yoga Association. 2011. "State Regulation of Yoga Teacher Training." Accessed May 16, 2011. http://www.texyoga.org/en/news/50-state-regulation-of-yoga-teacher-training-facts-opinions-and-firsthand-experience.html.

Thatcher, Ron. 2008. *Selling Yoga: A Handbook for the Ultimate Yoga Business Professional.* Charleston, South Carolina: BookSurge Publishing

Tomlinson, John. 1999. *Globalization and Culture.* Chicago: University of Chicago Press.

Tulsiramji Maharaj, Pujyaji Sri. 1945. "A Message of Peace to a World full of Unrest." Prepared from his sermon delivered on June 9, 1945, Sardarshahar, Bikaner, India. Calcutta: Surana Printing Works.

Turner, Bryan S. 1997. "The Body in Western Society: Social Theory and its Perspectives." In *Religion and the Body,* edited by Sarah Coakley, 15–41. New York: Cambridge University Press.

Turner, Victor. 2008 [1969]. "Liminality and Communitas." *The Ritual Process: Structure and Anti-Structure.* New Brunswick: Aldine Transaction Press.

Tweed, Thomas A., and Stephen Prothero. 1999. *Asian Religions in America: A Documentary History.* New York: Oxford University Press.

United States Office of the Federal Register. 2012. "Registration of Claims to Copyright." *Federal Register: The Daily Journal of the United States Government,* June 22. Accessed February 1, 2013. https://www.federalregister.gov/articles/2012/06/22/2012–15235/registration-of-claims-to-copyright.

Urban, Hugh B. 2000. "The Cult of Ecstasy: Tantrism, the New Age, and the Spiritual Logic of Late Capitalism." *History of Religions* 39(3) (February): 268–304.

——. 2003. *Tantra: Sex, Secrecy, Politics, and Power in the Study of Religion.* Los Angeles: University of California Press.

———. 2005. "Osho, From Sex Guru to Guru of the Rich: The Spiritual Logic of Late Capitalism." In *Gurus in America,* edited by Thomas A. Forsthoefel and Cynthia Ann Humes, 147–168. New York: State University of New York Press.

———. 2006. *Magia Sexualis: Sex, Magic, and Liberation in Modern Western Esotericism.* Los Angeles: University of California Press.

Vallely, Anne. 2002. *Guardians of the Transcendent: An Ethnography of a Jain Ascetic Community.* Toronto: University of Toronto Press.

Van Gennep, Arnold. 1965 [1908]. *The Rites of Passage.* London: Routledge & Kegan Paul.

Vanita, Ruth. 2003. "The Self is Not Gendered: Sulabha's Debate with King Janaka." *National Women's Studies Association Journal* 15(2): 76–93.

Vasudeva, Somadeva. 2012. "The Transport of the Haṃsas: A Śākta Rāsalīlā as Rājayoga in Eighteenth-Century Benares." In *Yoga in Practice,* edited by David Gordon White, 242–254. Princeton, NJ: Princeton University Press.

Viswanathan, Gauri. 2003. "Colonialism and the Construction of Hinduism." In *Blackwell Companion to Hinduism,* edited by Gavin Flood, 23–44. Oxford: Wiley-Blackwell.

Vitello, Paul. 2010. "Hindu Group Stirs a Debate Over Yoga's Soul." *New York Times,* November 27. Accessed November 27, 2010. http://www.nytimes.com/2010/11/28/nyregion/28yoga.html.

Vivekananda, Swami. 1982 [1896]. *Raja Yoga: Conquering the Internal Nature.* New York: Ramakrishna-Vivekananda Center.

———. 1992 [1896]. *Raja Yoga,* in *The Complete Works of Swami Vivekananda.* Calcutta: Advaita Ashrama.

Wallace, Vesna. 2011. "Mahayana Insights into the Origins of Yoga and Tantra." "Contextualizing the History of Yoga in Geoffrey Samuel's *The Origins of Yoga and Tantra*: A Review Symposium." *International Journal of Hindu Studies* 15(3): 333–337.

Wanderlust Festival. 2011. *Wanderlust.* Accessed September 1, 2012. www.whistler.wanderlustfestival.com/home.

Weber, Max. 1963 [1922]. *The Sociology of Religion.* Translated by Ephraim Fischoff. Boston: Beacon Press.

Whicher, Ian. 2002–2003. "The World-Affirming and Integrative Dimension of Classical Yoga." *Cracow Indological Studies* 4–5: 619–636.

White, David Gordon. 1996. *The Alchemical Body: Siddha Traditions in Medieval India.* Chicago: University of Chicago Press.

———. 1999. "Tantric Sects and Tantric Sex: The Flow of Secret Tantric Gnosis." In *Rending the Veil: Concealment and Secrecy in the History of Religions,* edited by Elliot R. Wolfson, 249–270. Chappaqua, NY: Seven Bridges Press.

———. 2000. Introduction to *Tantra in Practice,* edited by David Gordon White. Princeton, NJ: Princeton University Press.

——. 2006. "'Open' and 'Closed' Models of the Human Body in Indian Medical and Yogic Traditions." *Asian Medicine: Tradition and Modernity* 2(1): 1–13.

——. 2009. *Sinister Yogis*. Chicago: University of Chicago Press.

——. 2012. Introduction to *Yoga in Practice*, edited by David Gordon White. Princeton, NJ: Princeton University Press.

Williams, Robert. 1963. *Jaina Yoga: A Survey of the Mediaeval Śrāvakācāras*. London: Oxford University Press.

——. 1965. "Haribhadra." *Bulletin of the School of Oriental and African Studies* 28(1): 101–111.

Williamson, Lola. 2005. "The Perfectibility of Perfection: Siddha Yoga as a Global Movement." In *Gurus in America*, edited by Thomas A. Forsthoefel and Cynthia Ann Humes, 147–168. New York: State University of New York Press.

——. 2010. *Transcendent in America: Hindu-Inspired Meditation Movements as New Religion*. New York: New York University Press.

——. 2014. "Stretching toward the Sacred: John Friend and Anusara Yoga." In *Gurus of Modern Yoga*, edited by Ellen Goldberg and Mark Singleton, 210–234. New York: Oxford University Press.

Willis, Paul. 1990. *Common Culture*. Milton Keynes: Open University Press.

Wilson, H. H. 1928. *Essays and Lectures, Chiefly on the Religion of the Hindus*. London: Trubner.

Wittgenstein, Ludwig L. 1953. *Philosophical Investigations*. Oxford: Blackwell.

Yeats-Brown, Francis. 1935. "Yoga for You," *Cosmopolitan*, April.

Yoga Alliance. 2013. "Yoga Alliance." Accessed October 10, 2012. http://yogaalliance.org.

Yoga Dork. 2012a. "Letter from John Friend to Anusara Yoga Teachers." Accessed March 7, 2012. http://www.yogadork.com/news/letter-from-john-friend-to-anusara-yoga-teachers/.

——. 2012b. "Running Timeline of Anusara Controversy." Accessed September 1, 2012. http://www.yogadork.com/news/running-timeline-of-anusara-controversy-updates-and-teacher-resignations/.

——. 2012c. "Update: John Friend on Reorganization, Letter from Newly-Appointed Anusara Inc., CEO." Accessed March 7, 2012. http://www.yogadork.com/news/update-john-friend-on-reorganization-letter-from-newly-appointed-anusara-inc-ceo/.

Yoga One. 2013. "Houston." Accessed February 23, 2013. http://yogaonehouston.com/teacher/?id=2.

Yoga Rocks the Park. 2014. "About." *Yoga Rocks the Park*. Accessed April 1, 2014. http://www.yogarocksthepark.com/about.html.

Yoga to the People. 2011a. "About YTTP: About Us." *Yoga to the People*. Accessed January 5, 2012. www.yogatothepeople.com/about-us/.

——. 2011b. "About YTTP: Mantra." *Yoga to the People*. Accessed January 5, 2012. www.yogatothepeople.com/about-us/mantra/.

———. 2011c. "About YTTP: YTTP Apparel." *Yoga to the People*. Accessed January 5, 2012. www.yogatothepeople.com/about-us/yttp-apparel/.

Young, Allan. 1980. "The Discourse on Stress and the Reproduction of Conventional Knowledge." *Social Science and Medicine* 14B: 133–146.

Zauberman, Gal. 2003. "The Intertemporal Dynamics of Consumer Lock-In." *Journal of Consumer Research* 30(3) (December): 405–419.

Index

CPSIA information can be obtained
at www.ICGtesting.com
Printed in the USA
BVHW031448291219
568041BV00002B/3/P